"Lynda Young cares deeply about children with cancer and their families. In this poignant book, her concerned passion shines through every page."

—**CECIL MURPHEY**, author or co-author of more than 100 books including the New York Times Best Seller, *90 Minutes in Heaven*

"Each year 12,000 children and teens are diagnosed with cancer. If you are a parent who has a child with cancer, this book is for you. You need not walk alone. Lynda Young brings you the benefit of hearing voices of others who have walked this road. It is truly a book of Hope."

—**GARY CHAPMAN**, PhD, author of *The Five Love Languages*

"Lynda T. Young and Chaplain Johnnathan Ward have written an extraordinary book that will be a valuable resource for every family member of a child diagnosed with cancer. It's filled with practical suggestions and inspirational encouragement, with a reminder that humor must always be an important part of making it through devastating circumstances. The true stories are heart touching, but the unique take-home value of this book consists of the comprehensive lists of 'what to do' during every stage of a child's journey through cancer. This book is the gift you will want to place in the hands of someone in your church or community who has a child diagnosed with cancer. I highly recommend it!"

—**CAROL KENT**, speaker and author of *A New Kind of Normal*

"Hope For Families of Children with Cancer is written with gentle sensitivity and compassion. It is also a practical, down-to-earth guide offering strength, faith, and direction for families who are walking through this traumatic and frightening experience. The book is emotional, yet informative and beautifully articulate."

—**DIANA L. JAMES**, speaker, radio host, and author of the *Bounce Back* series and other books.

"Traversing the emotional roller coaster of a child's unexpected illness is a parent's greatest struggle. I know. I've been there. From the heart-pounding moment of the diagnosis through the twists and turns of unfamiliar terms, treatments, and trials, Lynda Young and Chaplain Ward gently and compassionately address the frequently asked question, 'What do I do now?' Parents, grandparents, and friends of toddlers to teens will find this book packed with real-life situations, practical helps, nuggets of humor, and comforting spiritual encouragement. I highly recommend it!"

—**FRAN CAFFEY SANDIN**, RN, BSN, author of *See You Later, Jeffrey* and *Touching the Clouds: Encouraging Stories to Make Your Faith Soar*

"*Words of hope and encouragement, as well as guidance and practical advice, are beautifully woven together in this easy-to-read resource. Thoughts and feelings from parents who have walked the childhood cancer road offer comfort and understanding to those now facing the overwhelming journey that no one ever wants to take. If this book had been available a few years ago when one of my children was born with cancer I would have kept it by my side . . . what a blessing it will offer to those who need hope during a time that feels so confusing and out of control.*"

—**STUART SWEITZER**, A Place Called Hope, Inc., Baltimore, MD

"*God never shuts a door without opening a window! This book will help many windows open in the lives of our families. It is a wonderful resource for families of children with cancer.*"

—**SHEILA MOORE**, MD, Medical Director St Jude Affiliate Clinic/Baton Rouge

"*I've been associated with several books for parents of children with life-threatening diseases—and saw my brother and his wife struggle as their eight-year-old son battled cancer.* Hope for Families of Children with Cancer *provides the emotional and spiritual support parents need, with stories of families doing battle with their child's cancer revealing the family dynamics. While families' experiences differ, it's amazing how similar reactions tend to be—and this book holds up a mirror that builds understanding and may well help save marriages and prevent the alienation of siblings that so often happens.*"

—**LES STOBBE**, literary agent

"*[Dear Lynda and Johnnathan,] I found the book so very insightful in the cancer journey. I have many times seen just what you are describing. You have done a very excellent job in capturing the emotional and spiritual dimensions of the journey in the world of child hood cancer. This is a journey that is the nightmare of any parent, but one traveled hundreds of times each week. I would recommend this book to any medical caretaker as well as a family just beginning. I would also recommend it for anyone who is attempting to help families in their journey. Again this is an excellent work.*"

—**DANNY L. CAVETT** MLS Director of Pastoral Care/EAP, Oklahoma City University Medical Center

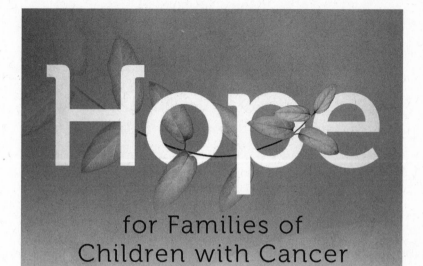

Hope

for Families of Children with Cancer

Lynda T. Young

and Johnnathan R. Ward

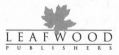

LEAFWOOD
PUBLISHERS

HOPE FOR FAMILIES OF CHILDREN WITH CANCER

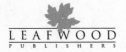

Copyright 2011 by Lynda T. Young and Johnnathan R. Ward

ISBN 978-0-89112-289-0
LCCN 2011022952

Printed in the United States of America

Scripture taken from the New King James Version. Copyright © 1982 by Thomas Nelson, Inc. Used by permission. All rights reserved.

LIBRARY OF CONGRESS CATALOGING-IN-PUBLICATION DATA
Young, Lynda T.
 Hope for families of children with cancer / by Lynda T. Young and Johnnathan R. Ward.
     p. cm.
 Originally published: Snellville, Ga. : Kindred Press, c2008.
 Includes bibliographical references and index.
 ISBN 978-0-89112-289-0 (pbk.)
 1. Cancer--Popular works. 2. Cancer in children--Psychological aspects--Family relation-ships--Popular works 3. Cancer--Patients--Family relationships--Popular works. I. Ward, Johnnathan. II. Title.
 RC281.C4Y678 2011
 618.92'994--dc23

                                                                    2011022952

Cover design by Thinkpen Design, LLC
Interior text design by Sandy Armstrong

Leafwood Publishers is an imprint of
Abilene Christian University Press
1626 Campus Court
Abilene, Texas 79601

1-877-816-4455
www.leafwoodpublishers.com

          11 12 13 14 15 16 / 7 6 5 4 3 2 1

Cancer Is So Limited . . .

It cannot cripple love.
It cannot shatter hope.
It cannot erode faith.
It cannot destroy peace.
It cannot wipe out confidence.
It cannot kill friendship.
It cannot suppress memories.
It cannot silence courage.
It cannot invade the Soul.
It cannot steal Eternal Life.
It cannot conquer the Spirit.
It cannot lessen the power of Resurrection.

Anonymous Author

Dedication

To the families, children, and medical staff whose hope cuts through the darkness of this cancer journey.

To my husband, Dr. John Young, who has set a standard in cancer research for over forty years, and encouraged the writing of this book—which seemed to take me forty years.

To those who've prayed through the writing of this book and prayed for those who would read it. Only in heaven will all those prayers be known.

And most importantly, to the One our hope is in.

Contents

Thank You

Lynda Young

I love looking back to see God's open doors—especially those I didn't even know existed. Thank you Les Stobbe, the literary agent who walked this road with his family, for suggesting I write the book on my heart for families of children with cancer. Your encouragement began the process.

Thank you Chaplain Johnnathan Ward. I am grateful for your sage advice, your prayer support, and the time you carved out of your demanding schedule as you served and encouraged others in the trenches. It was a privilege to work with you to craft a book to touch the hearts of the hurting.

Thank you Cec Murphy for your valuable mentoring writing sessions and for all the time you give to new writers.

Thank you to those who provided proofreading and encouragement. And thank you to those who prayed for the writers and readers. You know who you are—and you have done eternity's work.

Hope

Cancer. Heart disease. Chronic conditions such as autistic spectrum, sickle cell, diabetes, mental handicaps, organ transplants, and other diseases—all are devastating—but when they happen to a child they take our breath away. How do we go on? Surely, the only way forward is with hope.

Devastating diagnoses send families reeling, plunging them into the world of the *new normal*: new places (specialists and hospitals), new people, and new procedures. Lives are changed forever. Fortunately, fellow travelers who've been there are willing to help guide the way through unfamiliar territory. Medical professionals and hospital volunteers also come alongside weary caregivers. That support is vital as primary caregivers try to balance the needs of their sick child with the needs of their family (set-aside spouses and the child's seemingly invisible siblings) and themselves.

My marriage of forty years to a cancer researcher, and my own work as a volunteer in a local children's hospital, eventually led me to write *Hope for Families of Children with Cancer*. But as I worked on it people questioned me: "Why is the book just for cancer families when there are so many diseases that families face?" And they were right.

Hope for Families of Children on the Autistic Spectrum (Leafwood Publishers 2011) and *Hope for Families of Children with Congenital Heart Defects* are the next books to be released in the You Are Not Alone book series. Each book includes encouraging short stories, refreshing helpful hints, and comforting inspirational scriptures. All families need rays of sunshine to provide hope in the darkness. Everyone needs to know, as they walk in unfamiliar territory, they are not alone.

Circumstances may appear to wreck our lives and God's plans, but God is not helpless among the ruins.

—Eric Liddell, Olympian

God's Coincidence?

Childhood cancer is not a journey anyone chooses—not children, parents, family, friends, not anyone. I haven't walked this path, but I've been privileged to walk with those who have as I've volunteered at a children's hospital schoolroom in Atlanta. Volunteering has taken care of my retired-teacher needs. I missed those moments when things clicked and a child got it. Even more importantly, I've been blessed with God's coincidences, those moments when things clicked and *I* got it.

That's what happened one morning in the schoolroom. One of the teachers said, "Lynda, there's a seven-year-old girl in room 356 that needs bedside tutoring. She's in isolation—in for a bone marrow transplant (BMT). Do you have time to go?" I did have time, so I stepped into the elevator and prayed my usual quick prayer: *Please use me, Lord.* Third floor chimed, the doors slid open, and I headed down the hall.

I stopped at the closed isolation doors and hit the entry button. My shoes clicked down the short hall, four rooms on each side; carts stacked with disposable masks, gowns, and gloves leaned against the wall. I turned to the metal hand-washing sink and stepped on the floor pedal. The cool water mingled with soap and sloshed over my hands.

How long did they say to do this? Twenty seconds?

I grabbed the paper towels, tossed them into the trash, and turned to 356.

Each time I stood outside the BMT rooms, I was apprehensive. I always wondered if I could be of any help in these extremely difficult situations. I knocked gently on the door.

A muffled voice said, "Come in."

I pushed the door open slowly, "Hi, I'm Lynda Young from the schoolroom, here to help Danielle."

The mom waved me in from across the room as she finished brushing her teeth at the sink. "I'm Hedy. Sorry, I just have to get this done when I can."

I walked over to Danielle propped up in bed, her black hair pulled back in a red kerchief. Purple and blue paints, paper, scissors, and pipe cleaners filled her tray table.

"What a cool butterfly picture," I said.

She smiled wanly.

"Do you feel like doing any schoolwork?"

"I just want to paint."

I glanced around the room at photos of two beaming little sisters, floating butterfly-shaped balloons tied to the IV pole, and art projects tacked to the walls—making the room home 24/7. On Hedy's chair, her well-worn Bible laid open.

Hedy leaned over her single bed/sofa and folded the sheets, "Here, sit down." I sat down and shifted pillows against the wall for comfort. She shoved her books to the side and sat at the other end of the bed. She told me Danielle's cancer had returned after a four-year remission and they fit the protocol in Atlanta, so they moved from Miami, Florida. Danielle was scheduled for a bone marrow transplant from one of her sisters.

"My husband's new job fell through when we arrived," she told me. Unfortunately, her story continued downhill from there, including losing the down payment on their house and their car being wrecked. "You have to laugh not to cry. The storage unit has charged four times the amount they had quoted, so they're holding our furniture hostage. All we have is in the suitcases we brought from Florida."

She told all that without bitterness, just with exhaustion and a faint smile. "I know God is in control, but we're so weary."

Danielle's eyes slowly closed as the IV pain medications took effect. She pushed the tray to the side of the bed and snuggled against her pillows.

"I'm going to be praying for Danielle, and you and your family," I whispered.

"Thank you so much. How can I pray for you?"

For me?

> ### God's Promise
> Greater love has no one than this, than to lay down one's life for his friends.
> —John 15:13

"Well, as a matter of fact, our son and his family are going through a rough time. They've just moved from Missouri to Wisconsin, and when they got there, the house they were going to rent was a shambles. So, the six of them have been living in a motel room for weeks."

"They do need prayer!"

"I know it isn't anything compared with your situation."

"But it's tough for them."

A few minutes later, I left the room, I had no idea how this woman and child would affect my life. Since 2002, we've shared Hedy's reoccurring struggles, deep valleys, and God's provisions.

God's coincidence? I got it.

Connections

There are levels of friendship. Some people you know for years but share only the surface of life. With others, you share more and go deeper. But then there are those with whom you share a crisis—and you dive deep fast.

In this book, parents from all over the country (and overseas) share their stories and connect through their universal crisis: childhood cancer. They've shared their journeys with us in this book hoping to connect and come alongside you, the reader. Some of the stories are compilations of several similar experiences. In the stories, unless otherwise noted, the "I" telling the story is Lynda. Again, I haven't walked this difficult path, but I am privileged to share these journeys with you.

On your journey, keep your eyes open for those with whom you'll share struggles, deep valleys, and God's provisions. Don't miss these opportunities; and more importantly, don't miss him. You're not alone.

When a train goes through a tunnel and it gets dark, you don't throw away the ticket and jump off. You sit still and trust the engineer.

—Corrie ten Boom

2

I'm Sorry to Tell You This . . .

"Cancer was the last thing we ever expected." We wonder how many times we've heard parents say, "She's only a child. You don't expect children to get cancer." However, each year more than 12,000 children and adolescents are diagnosed with cancer, added to the 270,000-plus survivors of childhood cancer. This may seem like a small percentage compared to the millions of children twenty and younger in the United States, but not to parents walking this path with their child.

"What do you mean 'a small percentage'?" Bob said as he reeled from his daughter's leukemia diagnosis. "The percentage doesn't matter when it's your child. I've never felt so helpless or alone."

Helpless, alone, overwhelmed—all are normal feelings—you aren't losing your mind, it just feels that way. Many cancer families label this the new normal as their lives adjust to new people, new places, and new protocols.

When you hear, "I'm sorry to tell you this—your child has cancer," your life splits into two parts: life before the cancer, and life with cancer. Each day demands new decisions, presents new challenges, and draws out perseverance that you never knew you had. Each day may bring you to the point of exhaustion, but you keep going.

"But you'll also experience kindness from the hospital staff," a mom said, "nurses who plan ahead to give nausea meds before your child goes to the hospital schoolroom, or a smile from the lady who cleans your hospital room floor. Or a parent who takes time to give you financial information they discovered and then hands you a book of parking garage passes."

Whether you've just begun this journey, or have persisted for weeks, months, or years, we want to encourage you with stories from your fellow travelers. Others have gone before you and, unfortunately, others will follow. Every childhood cancer story is unique, but all share similar struggles, trials, and hopes.

As a childhood cancer family, your life has been split in two parts. This book brings hope for that second part. You are not alone.

When the Bevins family approached that second part, cancer was the last thing they ever expected.

One Family's Story

Before the Diagnosis: Approaching the Tunnel

Ten-year-old Alex ran wildly at recess. As he raced, his friend Derrick elbowed him. They rolled over and over as each scrambled for the ball. That evening Alex began to limp.

"What's wrong with your leg?" Judy, his mom, asked.

"It kinda hurts."

Over the next few weeks, the limping continued. A visit to his pediatrician hadn't given an answer to the problem. The doctor called Judy to bring Alex in again. He said, " . . . and this time, bring your husband."

The next day, Judy checked Alex out of school at noon while John waited in the car and read his office's text messages.

"My friends all gave me high-fives 'cause I got to leave early," Alex said as they headed out the main door.

An hour later, Alex sat on the paper-covered table in the doctor's office; his thumbs quickly manipulated the DS. Thirty minutes passed.

Judy glanced at her watch before she turned to John, "How long till the doctor comes back?"

Without looking up, Alex mumbled, "It's no big deal."

After another fifteen minutes, the door opened. "Sorry it took so long. We've gotten the results from the tests, and I'm going to send you to another doctor tomorrow for a consult."

"Another doctor? What's wrong?" Judy asked.

"It's just a sore leg," Alex said.

"Let's wait and see what Dr. Wyatt says; I want us to be sure."

"Am I going to have to miss another football practice?"

Smiling, the doctor said, "I don't think so. Your parents can go see him without you."

Alex's thumbs continued to fly, "Cool."

The Diagnosis: Sucked into Darkness

Another doctor, the pediatrician said. A pediatric oncologist is certainly another doctor, all right. Judy gulped the last drops of lukewarm coffee from the Styrofoam cup. Staring into space, she pinched pieces from the rim. Every few minutes she glanced at the clock above the receptionist's window and checked it against the time on her watch. The nurse called another family back.

John thumbed through last month's sports magazine. Judy picked up the *Better Homes* magazine, glanced at the cover, tossed it on the table, and then stared into space again.

"Bevins family?" called the nurse.

Jarred back to reality, Judy grabbed John's arm. They stood, and she tossed the crunched cup into the trashcan. Her heart pounded as they followed the nurse down the hall. Judy clutched John's arm and leaned closer to his side. He slid his hand to cover her trembling hands.

They passed examining rooms on each side. A door opened, and a bald toddler ran into the hall. Her mother quickly followed and swung her up into her arms.

"You'd think I'd be used to this and watch the door," she said, and went back into the room toting the wiggly child.

A child with cancer? Our child? Judy's nails dug into John's sleeve. *Is that what Alex will look like?*

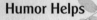

Humor Helps

Waiting rooms breed Styrofoam cups.

"It's okay," John whispered and kissed her forehead.

. The nurse knocked on the doctor's half-opened door and set Alex's file on his desk.

"Come in," he said and motioned them into the room.

"I'm Dr. Wyatt, please sit down. I've heard Alex is quite the football player."

"That's his whole life, and racing his bike down our steep hill," John said.

> **Every Moment**
>
> While you're waiting on answers from God your Father, value every moment. Don't live in the future while today is ticking away. He desires to have an active presence in your life each day.

The doctor's warm smile and small talk eased the tension . . . somewhat. He adjusted his bifocals and scanned the last page. "We have the test results, and I'm sorry to tell you this—Alex has cancer."

John tightened his grip on Judy's hand. "Oh, my God," he stammered. "There has to be a mistake."

"There have to be more tests you can run, right?" Judy asked.

"We've run all we can."

"You must have overlooked something."

Dr. Wyatt shook his head.

"But how did this happen?"

"Why did this happen to Alex? He's so healthy!"

"What else can we do?"

Shocked responses poured out of them, and none of the doctor's answers relieved their fears as he explained Alex's type of cancer. Scary, unfamiliar words echoed in the room: chemotherapy, radiation, prognosis.

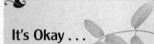

It's Okay . . .

It's okay to cry—tears clear our vision. Dads, that's for you, too.

Dazed, John and Judy just stared at the doctor's face.

"Here are the next steps . . ."

His mouth is moving, but what's he saying? Judy wondered.

"I know you won't remember what I've said, so here it is on paper." He handed them a folder.

Judy took the folder from his hands, and they slowly stood. Suddenly Judy's knees buckled; both men grabbed her arms to steady her.

"This is such a hard time," continued the doctor, "but we'll be in touch with you tomorrow."

"I don't know how you do this job," John said. "But thank you." John took Judy by the arm and they walked to the receptionist's window.

"We need to schedule your appointments," the receptionist said.

Judy dug to the bottom of her purse. "Where's my calendar? I know it's here," she said to the receptionist. *It's just a pulled muscle . . .*

"Take your time," the nurse said, sliding the tissue box toward her.

Behind her, John sniffled. At that, tears streamed down her face.

"Just keep the box," the nurse said, patting Judy's hand.

Walking outside, they shielded their eyes from blinding sunlight and wondered how it could be so bright.

Single Caregivers: Alone in the Tunnel

"It's bad enough when you've heard those awful words while someone else is with you, but as a single parent sitting there all by yourself—I can't even describe it. You feel totally alone," a single caregiver said.

The devastating diagnosis can leave single caregivers feeling besieged. How do they split their limited time? At work? With their child in the hospital? With the siblings at home?

"There wasn't enough of me, and no one else to lean on. Money got tighter, I couldn't pay bills, and previous problems with my insecurities and fears shot to the surface."

As a single caregiver, you may feel as if everything lands on your shoulders. (You might flip over to Chapter Seven for helpful suggestions that deal with common problems of all caregivers.)

"I envy families who have support from other people. I'm in this by myself with my sick grandchild. Where do I go for help?" As a single caregiver, you carry the weight of family decisions, but you need to share that load with others who come alongside. The following are suggestions from others who have walked

> ### God's Word in the Tunnel
>
> Dear caregivers, whatever your situation, hold on to this truth: God cares about you and your precious child. You can't be God for your children, but you can hand them over to him. These are his words: "When you pass through the waters, I *will be* with you; And through the rivers, they shall not overflow you. . . ."
>
> —Isaiah 43:2
> He will be there.

this journey as a single caregiver—those who understand how you feel.

- Don't isolate yourself. Seek and join support groups for single caregivers at the hospital or online. They understand your difficult journey. Church groups and friends may not understand the difficulties, but they can provide emotional, physical, and spiritual help. Your time is limited and it's hard to carve out the hours for support, but make this a priority. Not only will this benefit you, but it will benefit your child as you are strengthened and encouraged.
- When your child was first admitted to the hospital, you probably received a notebook overflowing with information. If you can't find financial resource help, ask the hospital social worker to lead you to the assistance you need.
- Try to establish consistent daily routines. Even small amounts of time set aside can balance the stress of hospital, home, and work. A quick story before bedtime, a drive-through meal together, or a telephone call at a specific time may bring security for you and your family—something to look forward to.
- Encourage consistent discipline of your child and their siblings by those who help you take care of them. Everyone needs to know how you want things done. It relieves second-guessing.
- Treat kids like kids, not a substitute for an adult partner. It's easy to put the oldest child into an adult role when you're exhausted and need help.

- Keep communication lines open with others through e-mails, CarePages, or CaringBridge sites (see Resource Two).

Reactions in the Tunnel

After the devastating diagnosis, most family members express these feelings:

- "Oh, God! I feel like I've been punched in the stomach."
- "I'm walking through a fog, sort of an out-of-body experience."
- "This can't be happening to my child." (shock)

But the real differences arise in the next steps as parents or care-givers seek to cope with an overwhelming situation. One mom said, "When we first heard the diagnosis, my husband, Tom, searched the Internet for days trying to find more information. I collapsed in tears trying to deny the diagnosis. How could we react so differently? He's *our* child."

The truth is that cancer changes the dynamics of the family. All members are still who they are, but their personalities become intensified. Weaknesses become more obvious, and strengths are often taken to the extreme in an attempt to cope. Unfortunately, even good things can be overdone.

Some parents forage for information by searching the Internet. Some try to find help via chat rooms and support groups. Some shut down emotionally, and others cry or talk uncontrollably. Others' reactions may not make sense to you, but they make sense to the reactor.

We all respond differently to stress. In Tom's case his strength, searching for information, helped them make wise treatment decisions. His calm demeanor and task-oriented plans brought some control over the uncontrollable situation as they met with doctors. He compartmentalized his feelings and focused on his child's drastic diagnosis.

However, Tom lost himself in the search for information and distanced himself from the family and his wife's emotions. His wife, Janet, felt that he pulled away and shut down when she needed him most.

By contrast, she turned outward, to others, communicating with hugs, tears, and talking to her network of friends and family. That network was already in place. Janet had reached out through her strengths to help others in need over the years. Now she needed much in return.

Unfortunately, Tom was unable to express the emotions she needed from him, so she shut him out. Neither appreciated the strengths the other brought to the marriage, nor understood the other's behavior. Both ran on empty emotionally, with little to give the other as they dealt with the daily care of their sick child.

Initial behavior that starts out as a reaction to the shocking diagnosis can harden into a pattern. Sometimes each spouse's coping mechanisms can result in the two parents pulling in opposite directions, trying to balance one another out. Take a few minutes to sit and talk face to face. Each ask, "What one thing can I do to help you today?" Then listen, and try to do what was asked. These few minutes invested in

Reactions

Others' reactions may not make sense to you, but they make sense to the reactor.

34

each other will bring long-lasting rewards in filling those drained emotional tanks.

A great resource is *The Five Love Languages: How to Express Heartfelt Commitment to Your Mate,* as well as the other books in the Five Love Languages series. In them Gary Chapman gives new insights on how we give and receive love.

One dad said, "My wife smothers our daughter, so I have to balance it by being objective."

His wife's response? "'Smothers?' She needs all my attention, and I intend to give it to her . . . "

Each partner pulled in the opposite direction trying to balance the situation and the result was an emotional tug-of-war. This is the kind of tension that builds up and hangs like invisible gas in the home. Then all it takes is the least spark—a harsh tone or rolling of the eyes—to ignite an explosion.

Such a volatile atmosphere makes it nearly impossible to make the excruciating decisions that cancer requires. The explosions can shake the entire family, and communication can further break down.

Take time to think about the coping mechanisms you are using. What about your spouse and the rest of your family? How is each person coping? Are empty emotional tanks creating a tug-of-war?

How do you drop your end of the rope in this tug-of-war and come alongside them? When your spouse or other family members are frustrating you, take time to consider that they, too, are just trying to cope with an overwhelming situation. They may not cope in the same way as you, but they're trying to make their way through. Ask God to show you their strengths, and then tell them you appreciate who they are and what they do. It will be like cool water poured on parched ground.

Talking in the Tunnel

Some parents are able to talk about their child and their feelings. The open dialogue brings them closer together. However, many parents can't do this. They *can* discuss treatment plans with the doctors and carpool schedules with neighbors, but they fill every moment to avoid the main issue—their feelings about their child's diagnosis and treatment.

"Why didn't we talk about our child and our feelings?" one CK's mom said. "If we talked about it, it made it more real and the pain seemed twice as bad. But we also ended up feeling abandoned by each other. We finally opened up and what a relief to get those fearful feelings out, and we continued talking about it later." That mom had a few suggestions:

- Pray together each day about the situation. Ask God to lead your decisions and to give you strength.
- Express your fears openly to each other.
- Watch for opportunities to encourage each other when you're down.

Another mom said, "Talk and pray each day? I don't even have time to take a fast shower."

Sound familiar? When you think you have the least time for talking and praying, it's when you need it most. Don't let communication lapses continue. Every day that passes makes it more difficult to do. It may feel risky to reach out. You may find it easier to begin with a question. Ask your spouse about his or her

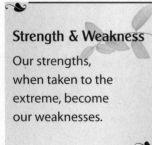

Strength & Weakness

Our strengths, when taken to the extreme, become our weaknesses.

fears, and be sure to listen respect-fully. Don't judge and don't write off those fears as if they're not important.

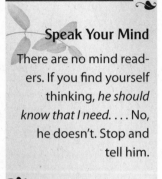

Speak Your Mind

There are no mind read-ers. If you find yourself thinking, *he should know that I need.* . . . No, he doesn't. Stop and tell him.

As you think about bridging the communication gap, you may feel fearful that you'll be rebuffed by others who don't see the need for talk-ing about the situation. It may seem easier to avoid the pain and hold your feelings inside, but it's worth taking the chance as walls come down and you connect emotionally with each other.

"I didn't know if we'd ever talk again, at least not on a deep level," a mom said. "We'd been dealing with our child's cancer for three years, and one night my hus-band collapsed and sobbed. We sat on the sofa and I cradled him in my arms. That 220-pound man who'd been my rock crumbled. And the rest of the night we talked, cried, and prayed. I wish he'd been able to do that in small steps each day or week—not in one huge meltdown. We've done better since then, and we try to make a 'date,' even in the hospital cafeteria over coffee, to say how we're feeling."

This journey is a marathon, not a dash, and daily decisions affect our relationships for the future. By choosing to encourage one another, fill emotional tanks, and draw together, each step of the journey can at least be a little lighter. Choose to see whether you're discouraging your partner in some way or draining your partner's emotional tank. If you don't make active choices to draw together, you may find yourselves drifting apart—even far apart.

Let's look at some ways we can get our emotional tanks filled and how we can fill others' tanks for the journey.

Understanding Others In The Tunnel

Especially on this journey, communication is desperately needed with *all* the people in your life—family, friends, and hospital staff. Throughout this book, we refer to the You-niquely Made Personality Study, which highlights four basic personality types. (See Resource One for the whole study.) An understanding of personality types can help you enhance communication and fill others' empty emotional tanks. After a quick study of personality types, you may discover that your spouse, doctor, or sister isn't annoying you on purpose—it may simply be how they are "wired."

If you're interested, turn to Resource One. This will help you identify strengths and weaknesses (yours and others') and provide some ideas about how to handle those weaknesses.

God's Word on Partnership

Two *are* better than one, because they have a good reward for their labor.... And a threefold cord is not quickly broken.

—Ecclesiastes 4:9, 12

Depending on personality type, different factors drain and fill emotional tanks. The cancer journey is long and tanks need to be refilled—often. This study will help you do that.

The personality types in this study are color-coded because people connect emotionally to colors. Colors make it easier to remember the concepts—the outgoing Yellows, systematic Blues, driven Reds, and easygoing, shy Greens. One mom who read this study said, "That outgoing Yellow is so Kelly. That's why she's met everyone on the floor while I stayed in the room and hardly talked to our nurse. I feel more comfortable in mute-mode, I guess."

Most people say, "One of those colors is pretty much me, but I've also got a little of the others too." Everyone is a unique combination of colors—a blend. Your emotional gene pool comes from both sides of your family. Some people think that males or females are only certain colors.

One husband said, "Women are so much more emotional than men. My wife overreacts to everything." Of course, there are women and men in every color. One wife said, "My husband is the emotional one in our family. I'm the balanced one." Some people seem to be one-color people, while others are combinations of several, but everyone needs acceptance for who they are, appreciation for what they do, and encouragement to keep on being and doing in their unique way.

Using Your You-niquely Made Personality Study

As you read the You-niquely Made Personality Study in Resource One, jot notes in the margins to jog your memory of who needs what. When you're exhausted, "color-blindness" can cloud your perception. At those times it seems those optimistic Yellows aren't serious enough and don't follow through, the systematic Blues are too gloomy and nitpick every detail, the driven Reds don't care enough and boss others around, and the passive Greens don't show enough emotion and make napping an art form. Look for the *positives* in each person to clear up that "color-blindness." A single positive comment can beam a ray of hope even in the darkest tunnel, and everyone can use all the rays they can get.

Worry does not empty tomorrow of its sorrow; it empties today of its strength.

—Corrie ten Boom

What Do I Do Now?

New place—hospital.

New people—hospital staff.

New pain, new schedule, new procedures, new terminology, new problems, and none of it by choice.

"I'm trying to keep my head above water," a mom said, as she leaned against the wall outside her CK's room. "My brain is on overload with the new information and decisions I have to make. And my tears are right under the surface. Correction, here they come." She sighed and dabbed her already red-rimmed eyes. "I'm faced with my daughter's questions and fears, and I can't even handle my own. How can I know what to tell my daughter?"

To tell or not to tell is one of the first issues that parents face after a cancer diagnosis. For many parents, the first inclination is

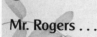

Mr. Rogers . . .

As Mr. Rogers said, "If it's mentionable, it's manageable." But first it has to be mentioned.

not to tell their child about the diagnosis. That instinct is a protective one, and it's understandable. But your child is probably going to hear it somewhere, and it's better if it comes from you. If you aren't open and honest, your child may think, "If Mom didn't tell me the truth about this, what else is she lying about?" You want to be the one in charge of telling your child. You don't want him overhearing it from someone else, especially if that someone else is another child with a wealth of misinformation.

Make time to sit with your child and explain on his level what is happening. Emphasize that you are telling the truth. Discuss how you and your family will work together with the doctors and nurses on the ways you will help him. You might say something like this: "We're all a team, and we as a family want to cooperate with the doctors and nurses so they can give you the best treatment possible."

Some parents reject telling their child because of the child's age. Parents of preschoolers may think, she's young and if I don't tell her, she'll just adjust. But that is simply not so. In fact, young children may imagine things are even worse than the truth. We've encountered adult survivors of childhood cancer who have told us that their parents didn't tell them the truth. At that time, that was all the parents knew to do—or *could* do. What the child thought was happening was quite different from what was actually going on. One survivor told us, "Parents didn't tell you things years ago. It wasn't talked about. I hope parents are better at that now."

Children believe the world revolves around them and may feel that they cause everything that happens. Educator Rudolf Dreikurs said, "Children are often excellent observers but poor interpreters." They observe everything but their understanding is immature. They may talk like small adults, but they don't have life experiences to evaluate what is happening. They need your adult wisdom and guidance.

As you consider what to say and how to say it, remember that you know your child's personality and moods better than anyone. You and your partner are also the most trusted people in your child's life.

Your child depends on you for honesty. Be honest right from the start, and in a gentle way give the information needed and appropriate for his understanding. This, of course, will depend on your child's age and personality.

One of the most important things to say is, "We're in this together." If he continues hearing these magical words from you, then he feels like part of the solution, having some control over an uncontrollable situation. If all the family shares the burden, it makes it seem lighter for everyone.

You may feel that you don't have the strength or wisdom to have an honest discussion with your child, but you can ask for help. First, you can ask God. Here's a prayer starter for you: "Dear Father, please give me the wisdom and the words for this journey—each step and each day. Thank you for all the help you've given through fellow travelers and staff." Wisdom and words. He'll do that.

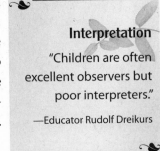

Interpretation

"Children are often excellent observers but poor interpreters."

—Educator Rudolf Dreikurs

45

> **Having Control**
>
> Give your child some control over an uncontrollable situation. You know how you're strengthened by having some control over a difficult situation.

Now let's look at some answers to common questions that CKs have about their situation. Perhaps that will give you a good launching point for talking with your child.

CK Questions

Your child may have many questions. What do you say? According to the National Cancer Institute, no matter what the cancer diagnosis, certain questions come up with almost all children. We've adapted some of the questions and answers from their website and included them here. (The National Cancer Institute's website www.cancer.gov is a wonderful resource.) These answers were provided by oncology professionals, but your answers should vary depending on the age and personality of your child. (Ages, stages, and personality traits are discussed in chapter four).

You might want to mark these questions and answers to have them ready—you never know when questions will arise. And, be prepared to work them into conversations with your child. Some children find it helpful if someone else opens the door to a conversation. You might simply say, "You may be thinking about . . . "

There are many resources available on the cancer journey, such as your child life specialist. They can give you words and appropriate times to discuss these issues with your child. Don't hesitate to ask any time you need help or support. Now, on to the questions and answers.

Why Did I Get Cancer?

Doctors don't even know. It wasn't anything that you or anyone else did.

Will I Get Well?

Cancer is a serious disease, but we have treatments and medicines that have gotten rid of cancer in many children, and the doctors and nurses are trying their best to cure your cancer, too.

What Will Happen to Me?

There are many types of childhood cancer and the doctor knows what medicines to use. Sometimes these medicines have side effects but the doctors have medicines to help those, too. (You might want to ask the doctors, nurses, or child life specialists how to explain side effects to your child—what to tell them and what will be done to help these situations.)

Why Do I Have to Take Medicine When I Feel Okay?

The medicine finds the bad cells, attacks them, and keeps them from coming back.

Did I Catch This from Anyone? Can Anyone Catch It from Me?

You can't catch it or give it to anyone else. It isn't contagious.

One Step at a Time

This is a long and difficult journey, and facing your child's honest questions is one of the many bumps in the road. Joshua, in the Old Testament, was on a difficult journey. He had led an entire nation, former slaves who'd been wandering in the desert for forty years, into fortified enemy territory. Overwhelmed by that challenge, he held on to these powerful words from God: " . . . Be strong and of good courage; do not be afraid, nor dismayed, for the LORD your God *is* with you wherever you go" (Josh. 1:9).

Your *wherever* may include chemotherapy, radiation, surgery, steroids, and heaviness while waiting for scans, tests, and results. As weakness, discouragement, and fear close in, hold on to these powerful words, " . . . the LORD your God *is* with you wherever you go."

Each day, ask God for strength and courage even, and especially when you think you can't keep going. Take a few minutes to take deep breaths—slowly in and out. When stressed, our breaths are shallow, but deep breaths relax the body. The next step is to take steps—one foot in front of the other. You may have to look down at your feet and say aloud, "One step at a time," but keep moving. You have to keep moving for your child.

As you continue to function each day (you get up and show up for life), ask God for wisdom about what to tell your CK and how to answer her questions. Rely on his help for you—and rely on his help for your child as you continue to put one foot in front of the other.

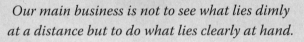

*Our main business is not to see what lies dimly
at a distance but to do what lies clearly at hand.*

—Thomas Carlyle

4

Caring for Your Unique Child

Whatever do thumbprints, snowflakes, and children have in common? They're unique—no two thumbprints, snowflakes, or children are exactly the same. You can't be "sort of" unique, says the dictionary. Unique is absolute, and your child is absolutely him- or herself—with a mixture of age, personality, and now diagnosis. Let's begin with the ages and stages your child goes through in their one-of-a-kind way.

Ages and Stages

We all know that children progress through stages as they mature. That doesn't change just because a child has cancer. CKs go through these stages too, but they have added variables due to cancer, treatments, and short- and long-term side effects.

Whether your CK is a baby, a teen, or somewhere in-between, you may want to read each of the age-group sections. Your family has expanded on this journey and now includes other parents and their CKs. Any advice you can share with other families regarding their children will be valuable.

Of course, the best advice is what you already know. All children—whatever their age, whether sick or well—need love. They mainly want you to be there for them.

Infants and Toddlers

This age learns through their five senses, and they live in the now. "Ones" toddle (anywhere they can). "Twos" trample (anything in sight). As the toddler adds a hearty, "No!" he wields power over those big people who chase him, pull objects out of his mouth, and grab him as he heads for the stairs or street.

Each child has his own individual timetable when he will do things. However, two important characteristics develop during these years: curiosity and exploration. It's that running, climbing, and stuffing-everything-in-the-mouth phase.

Despite your exhaustion from corralling your toddler, take advantage of the times with your CK in the hospital, clinic, or at home. Rock her (if she'll hold still), read to her, look into her eyes, talk and sing to her. Children this age love music, and they think Mom or Dad's singing voice is great—no matter what.

"Jonah's biggest fear was being separated from us and we just didn't want to leave him alone, especially in the new place [the children's hospital]. We had to come to the hospital directly from our pediatrician's office—and we got there with only one diaper and a sippy cup in my purse. He clung to me and clutched my neck when the nurses came in and out of the room. He didn't know anyone except us; actually, we didn't know anyone either. I'm sure he felt our fear even though we kept saying, 'Everything's okay.'

"On top of that, they had to insert IVs and take blood to get him ready for tests. It hurt and he didn't know what was going on. He was thirsty, but we weren't allowed to give him anything to drink—so he just cried and cried. I handed him off to his daddy and slipped into the bathroom to cry too. I knew he needed to feel some control of something; so after the tests, this kind nurse brought in a different color sippy cup, and I could give him a choice of the green or red one."

The dad added, "As soon as his grandma got there, we had his blankie from home. He'd never have made it through the night without it. The nurses told us to turn down the lights in the room and keep noise at a minimum for him to be calmer. They even suggested playing music with a slow beat—like a heartbeat. I knew they dealt with this all the time, but when she said, 'If you're calmer, he will be too,' I wanted to say, 'But, I'm not sure we'll ever be calm again.'"

Three- to Six-Year-Olds

Three- to six-year-old children are concrete thinkers and link illness with specific actions. They believe if they do certain things, then certain things will follow. For instance, if you take medicines, you feel better. When other children this age learn of the CKs cancer, they may think they can "catch" it. And, the CK may think she can give it to others. The concept that cancer can't be "caught" needs to be explained by parents, teachers, coaches, and anyone who interacts with your child and other children around your child.

Let's Pray

Thank you, Lord, for this little one, who is "precious in your sight," as the song says. You do love the little children of the world. Please surround us here in this room with Your presence and peace. Amen.

Again, children this age feel that the world revolves around them and they are in control of what happens. Just because they may use some of the big words (the cancer jargon they pick up), it doesn't mean they know what it is and what it does. They need a lot of age-appropriate information and reassurance from adults. It is difficult to explain things to these concrete-thinkers, but remember to turn to your child life specialist for help. That's just what Tabitha's parents did. "Tabitha had just turned four, and when they told us to tell her as much as she could understand at four, it seemed strange. We simply said, 'The medicine in that bag goes through that tube into your body and it will help you.' We knew she didn't understand cancer, we didn't either, but the child life specialist gave us words to use. They told us to let her know the tests might hurt, but wouldn't hurt for long. And it was great how the nurses would rub salve where they needed to numb the pain," Tabitha's mom said.

"With so many procedures being done, we tried to keep our minds occupied with field trips to the playroom, the outside garden, cafeteria, and family library—anywhere out of the room for a while. One of our favorite places was the small aquarium on the first floor. We watched the fish peacefully swimming, and small children's reactions to those fish. A two-year-old boy came down the hall and spotted the fish tank. He ran up to it, slapped his hands against the glass, and screamed, 'Nemo! Nemo!' Everyone watching really needed that laugh and it made our four-year-old feel very grown-up. She talked about 'that baby' for the rest of the day."

"Even when Tabby talked about being 'big,' I could tell she was still scared," her grandmother said. "We hadn't seen her suck her thumb and whine since she was two. Her favorite toys and quilt from home have helped that some. Maybe if I sucked my thumb and whined, it'd work for me too."

One mom said, "My five-year-old spouts off the names of her meds to any medical student who comes in the room." This is her new world and her new words.

The main thing children this age want is love and attention from their parents. They can get upset when ignored, so be sure you're paying attention to your child and not just to her cancer. Children this age like to help adults, so give them opportunities to fold clothes, bring you something from another room, or help pack a lunch. Being needed and appreciated can help fill emotional spaces the chemo and treatments may have sapped.

Even young children can feel depressed if left out of activities with friends. A weak immune system, hospitalizations, and fatigue can take their toll on friendships. Also, if your CK spent time in a group of three friends before the cancer, you may want to invite the friends over one at a time. Because three friends (especially girls) tend to leave a third child out, it's easy for the CK to be that one. Inviting one playmate at a time helps eliminate that possibility.

Seven- to Eleven-Year-Olds

The world of a child in this age group is ever expanding to friends, teachers, and coaches who are important to them. Keep these people in the loop through calls and e-mails. People want to help. Let them know the best way to reach out to your child.

The CK wants to be "normal" and fit in with a group. Being different in any way—how she looks, aptitude in class, the ability to participate in playground games, or missing school—may bring on teasing. Be on the lookout for that, and ask others (teachers in particular) to do the same.

Children this age may deal with the question, "Why me?"

There can be a lot going on in the life of a child in this age group. School becomes more demanding. Involvement in sports or other activities usually begins during this time. Friends become more and more important. The "Why me?" question arises—again. Your child may be able to hold it together all day, but when she gets home to a safe place, she may be irritable or fall apart.

Whatever the reason for her irritability, continue to validate her feelings of frustration. Those feelings may stem from school, or treatments and side effects, or fights with a sibling. Again, the "Why me?" Empathy is important. You might say something like this: "You seem to be very frustrated (sad, weepy, angry) today. I bet you get tired of these tests (meds, not feeling well)." Your CK needs to know you're trying to understand how she feels and you think her feelings are valid. After a tough day, it may help if you suggest some things she might enjoy doing that weekend. Give your CK something to look forward to and provide some control in the situation.

Morning & Bedtime

Pray for your child and with your child each morning and before bedtime:
Lord, I place my child in your hands. Help him to feel your presence as I place myself in those same hands. Amen.

As a parent, you might be tempted to pull back at this time and not be too concerned with your child's activities and interests, but CKs need a place to channel their emotions and the energy they do have. Try to involve your CK in activities that tap into her natural talents and interests and watch her self-esteem soar. Some children make crafts (such as bracelets, purses, and key chains) or art projects to give to others or to sell. Others are into games, music, or sports. If you're not sure what your child's niche is, take this time to note what interests her and do what you can to encourage those interests.

> ### Prayers & Visits
> This is a tender age and children are receptive to your praying for them each day. A visit from the chaplain or someone from your church would mean a great deal.

"I've always been really into sports," stated eight-year-old Kurt. "And then one day I got this headache, and here I am in this hospital. My mom seems upset. But as long as I can still play soccer, I'm fine."

Kurt left the room to walk his laps around the nurse's station.

"He says he's fine, but he's becoming more clingy and quiet," his mom said. "We've told him that we won't leave him alone. Of course he says, 'That's no problem,' but he looks relieved when we say that we're staying anyway."

Dad added, "When we talked about the side effects of the chemo, like losing his hair, we tried to make it light, and I told him his brother and I were going to shave our heads at the same time if that happens. He really got a kick out of that. Of course, we know at this age, his friends are extremely important to him, but we still count too. He's worried that he won't be able to help his soccer team, but he's more afraid that his friends will forget him and not sit with him at lunch when he goes back to school. It's been a long time since I was eight, but I guess I remember some of those concerns."

Teens

Changes occur rapidly during the middle school years (ages twelve to fourteen). Hormones kick in, which affect their bodies *and* their emotions. Teens in good health experience a kaleidoscope of emotions and opinions that can vary from day to day. A teen grappling with a life-threatening illness may experience that kaleidoscope more intensely.

Many teens this age are quite empathetic; teens on a cancer journey may become even more so. Those friends who look past your CK's "differences" may become steadfast friends, so help your CK keep those friends in the loop with day-to-day happenings.

Two years ago, Donna's son, Trevor (age twelve), began painful, exhausting, dark days, lightened by friends "cutting school." Actually, they had permission to skip classes, and one friend came each day to pass the time with Trevor in the hospital as he underwent his chemo treatments.

Donna said, "Back at home in the afternoons, if Trevor was wiped out, they'd just hang out and wait for him to wake up. Then, they'd play games. Time goes by so much faster when it's shared."

Let's Pray

Dear Lord,

Please help my child to cope with all the variables in her life. Give us wisdom in sharing information with teachers, friends, and others on our journey. Help others to understand this unique time in my child's life. Amen.

Later, I talked to Trevor, and he beamed.

"Mom told you about my friends, right?"

"You all must be really close."

"They're great guys. One of them wanted to be with me when I heard the last beep."

"The what?"

"When the chemo bag's empty. He'd been there with me through lots of bags, and he said, 'I want to hear that last beep.' And when all the treatments were over, I even had an end of treatment party! I thought it was something to celebrate."

Trevor was fortunate to have such faithful friends. Be aware that it's not uncommon for some friends to back away from your CK (not knowing how to handle the situation). If that happens, your CK may withdraw. Keep your eyes open to the social impact of your CK's health situation and don't shy away from discussing it.

Like most teens, CKs don't want to be different from their friends. Look at how most teens dress and talk—just like their friends. Now add chemo and steroid side effects to those everyday teen pressures, and consider what your teen may be grappling with. If your teen is asking to stay home from school, try to glimpse the story behind the story. What's going on? Encourage school attendance as much as possible in order to keep up with work and stay connected with friends. Each middle school situation is unique and may be difficult to adjust to at best, much less with cancer. Ask for help when needed, with counselors and child life specialists. Your teen may need to talk through the various reactions they get from friends—positive and negative.

Whatever the age of your teen, encourage him or her to reach out to younger CKs who respond to the "big kids."

"Sometimes they relate to them better than the adult professional staff," a nurse said and smiled. This interaction gets teens outside themselves. The truth is that everyone needs to be needed—especially these teens whose world is flipped upside down.

As teens transition to high school (ages fifteen to eighteen), their world may become even more social. They also experience even greater concerns about appearance and hair. Those concerns may seem frivolous to adults when there's a devastating diagnosis in the picture, but that's the world of teens. Don't be surprised if you hear a teen say something like this: "I can take chemo, surgery, whatever—just not losing my hair." If and when your teen has to deal with that, involve their friends. Those friends can do a lot to infuse strength, which the chemo has depleted.

Here's a blurb from a typical teen CarePage: "Okay, I've got orientation on Monday, Tuesday is band practice, Wednesday go to clinic, and spinal tap on Thursday. Then hang out with friends on Friday." Clinic and spinal tap are just thrown into the mix of the week. The new normal.

Your teen is two people in one. One needs independence to fly, and the other needs the security of a nest in which to rest. Those conflicting needs can cause a lot of confusion for teens and their families. How often do you see a healthy teenage boy resting with his head on mom's shoulder? Not too often. But that's a common sight in oncology clinic waiting rooms.

Choking back tears, one mom said, "This should be a 'breaking away' time, and there he lies in the bed—all six feet of him. He's dependant on my feeding and dressing him. I'm not sure which one of us it's harder on."

Teens know what they're missing in life, and depression can quickly set in. Staff members and other teens can cut through walls teens may build, perhaps more easily than parents can. Support groups for these "almost" adults are valuable. Support groups are valuable for their parents too. This journey is difficult for both.

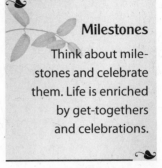

Milestones

Think about milestones and celebrate them. Life is enriched by get-togethers and celebrations.

Teens think in terms of symptoms and side effects—how they affect their everyday life and their future. They realize the importance of the treatments, even if they don't like them. However, at times, teens need to be reminded about the importance of their choices. Sometimes they will be tempted to go to an activity and not tell anyone (especially their mom) how sick they are. To them, a fever isn't worth missing a game, party, or some other fun event. Be sure someone from child life or a trusted nurse gets through to them about the importance of the long run. Even teens with cancer can feel indestructible; they need information from a trusted source so they can understand a spiked fever can drastically affect that long run.

Personality

Each age and stage brings so many changes; however, your child is always uniquely him- or herself—a blend of colors from that personality gene pool. As we've discussed, understanding personality types can help make this journey a little easier. Keep the types in mind as you deal with your CK and encounter others along the way. (Don't forget to turn to Resource One for more information.)

Yellows

Yellows not only see the glass half full—but overflowing! They want people around 24/7. They're emotional, but they're also resilient. They may be crying one minute, but they bounce back quickly—especially if there are people involved.

Adding steroids to these high-energy children? Tighten your grip as the roller coaster dives and jerks, but know that this too shall pass when the steroids are finished.

Encourage your Yellow's smile and outgoing personality and help them understand what a gift that is to others, especially in hospitals. Yellows can brighten everyone else's day, making twenty best friends on the first lap around the nurse's station.

Joseph was in remission and going strong when he turned sixteen. I knew the answer before I asked his mom the question: "How was Joseph's sixteenth birthday party?"

"I had to hold down the numbers to thirty of his very closest friends," she said smiling.

Again, Yellows need to receive hugs, positive comments, and attention—and they will give the same to others.

Let's Pray . . .

Dear Father,

Please give me your words to comfort and strengthen my teen's heart. Give him hope for each new day. Help me to let go as he grows. Help him and help me to view this journey through your eyes. Amen.

Blues

Blues tend to see the glass half empty. They feel pain more deeply and expect the worst will happen. "That last test hurt, so this one will for sure."

They like things done in order, so make charts that show progress.

Depending on your child's age, use smiley faces or other positive reinforcements after treatments, tests, and doctor and hospital visits. Let your child choose the stickers, realizing of course the length of time it will take in picking out the perfect ones.

Thank Blues for the ways they take care of things. "His room looks like my office, but more organized," one doctor whispered about his Blue patient. Having an organized room will fill any Blue's emotional tank.

They need to hear they've made a positive difference in others' lives. "Tyler, from down the hall, really appreciated the game you shared with him," a mom said. They also need to experience getting out of themselves and giving to others. Encourage that throughout their life, and especially now.

> ### Humor Helps
> You know you're a teen with cancer when . . .
>
> - The background on your phone is five, smiling bald people.
>
> - Your floor is covered with Tegaderm® papers.
>
> - You can't remember how to do long division but you can calculate, measure, and convert mls, mmls, and mgs of meds.
>
> From www.squirreltales.com
> —A support site for families of children with cancer.

Reds

Reds could care less if there's a glass, but if there is, they want to be in control of it. They direct others, the hospital staff included. "My daughter's been waited on hand and foot in the hospital and assumes that should continue at home. We had a battle royal getting her to pick up toys in her room. Fortunately, I'm as strong-willed as she," a Red mom said. "The good part is these strong-willed children persevere when others give up, and that's a plus in this world of cancer."

If a parent is an exhausted, low-energy Blue or Green, she may give in regarding rules with medication and other procedures.

"Everything seems like a major deal," a weary parent said.

Hang in there and choose your battles. Let the Red child have input and control when that's possible. They need that feeling. However, the battles you choose to win will give your strong-willed Red child boundaries and security.

Greens

Rather than experiencing the glass as half empty or as half full, Greens say, "What glass?"

Greens are sometimes overlooked because they don't demand attention as do the Reds and Yellows. If their parent is a self-starting Yellow or Red, a Green child simply follows their lead and instruction.

Because they're content to be inactive, Greens need to be prompted to get physical and mental exercise. Hours spent watching TV or sleeping can be counterproductive in the treatment program. Also, because Greens are accustomed to others making decisions for them, they need to be encouraged to take ownership in the treatment regimen. If you have a Green, discuss options with her and let her make those decisions (as appropriate to her age). Of course, if you're a Red parent, you'll find it difficult to abide by those decisions. However, the results will be good for her and good for you. She needs to take more control over her life, and you need to give it to her.

Helping Your Unique Child

We've talked about your unique child's age and personality. Now here are some more tools to add to your caregiver's toolbox in helping your CK.

Emotional Help

Whether your child is recently diagnosed or a veteran of the new normal, all children need stress relievers. Help them get the endorphins flowing to tell their brain they feel better. Read the section on endorphins in Chapter Seven.

Teach your child these stress-reducing techniques: deep breathing, squeezing a small stress ball, closing their eyes and imagining where they'd like to be, exercising (even wiggling toes and lifting their arms is a start), listening to their favorite music, and laughing. Child life specialists are great resources for helpful hints and ideas.

Providing a feeling of control over the situation can also help your child's emotional health. Depending on your child's age, your child should be part of the team that discusses their type of cancer, treatment, medicines, and side effects. You can also talk with your child about the timing of tests and treatments.

In an uncontrollable situation, even a calendar can help. You might say, "You pick out the calendar that you want to use so we can mark the days of doctor's visits, treatment, or tests." Most children feel as if they have some control while marking off the days.

However, don't tell younger children too far in advance about upcoming treatments; it may make them nervous because they have little understanding of time. How far in advance depends on the age and personality of your child. Make the calendar

> ### Spoiling Them
>
> "It is not giving children more that spoils them; it is giving them more to avoid confrontation."
>
> —John Gray

milestones a positive event for those sensitive Blues who've made an art form of worrying. Again, you know your child the best and what will work for her.

Discipline

Rules convey a sense of normalcy, and sticking by your family's rules will help your child. Of course, as we've seen, some children more easily comply with rules than others. Some, such as strong-willed Red children, are naturally more challenging—and can find ways to push the limits—even between bouts of throwing up!

After a cancer diagnosis, some parents wonder whether they should discipline their child. Some people say you can't spoil a cancer kid, and others say you can. Child life therapists tell parents, "If it was wrong before cancer, it's wrong during cancer." They have seen the effects of spoiling—effects on the child becoming self-absorbed, the parents' perceived guilt for never doing enough (emotional blackmail by CK), and siblings who crave attention and seldom get enough.

It's easier said than done, of course. Parents have a lot of reasons why they don't discipline or set limits. Here are a few:

- "It's hard to say no when your child has thrown up for hours."
- "When you're exhausted, it's just easier to give in."
- "I don't know which behaviors are related to the cancer and which aren't."

All these are valid reasons, especially when you're physically and emotionally drained. Take an attitude check—the child's attitude. Does he control decisions that you should be making? Is your child reacting one way in the hospital and another heading toward a favorite fast food place? Some parents say, "If I discipline my child, I'm afraid he won't love me as much."

This isn't about your child filling your needs. This concerns your child needing boundaries (rules) that only you can give. Rules give security and a sense of normalcy, whether he realizes it or not. When the rules remain the same even though the situation has changed, you are sending the message that things are sort of normal.

Do you think the demanding child, usually a controlling Red, whose room has more toys than the hospital gift shop will curb expectations when you go home? If a child can get anything she wants in the hospital, why not continue that at home, school, with grandparents, whomever they're with, and wherever they are?

"No one wants to be around a spoiled child, cancer kid or not," a parent said. That's especially true for the child's siblings who often feel left out. "I wish I had cancer so I get all that stuff," a CK's sibling told her mom. "But you see how sick he is," her mom said. When you're a six-year-old sibling, that explanation doesn't compute, you only see all the stuff.

So what happens next? "To even things out, we've tried to give the

Waiting . . .

Where do you get the wisdom and strength for each day? "Wait on the LORD; Be of good courage, And He shall strengthen your heart; Wait, I say, on the LORD!"

—Psalm 27:14 Wait on him.

siblings equal gifts. We have several other children and this is breaking us! Where does this stop?" a mom asked.

"I guess it stops when we say so," the dad responded under his breath.

Whether your child has siblings or he's an only child, gifts are appropriate—just make sure they aren't overdone. Need help with appropriate discipline, and how much gift giving to do? Talk to your child life specialist and other professionals. They've seen it all and are valuable resources.

Spiritual Help

Because of this demanding journey, parents may only focus on the physical and emotional parts of the child. Don't neglect the part you can't see—the spiritual. Praying (simply talking to God) with your child each day connects your CK with him. Your child learns to walk, talk, and become a person by mimicking you. Keep in mind that much is caught, not taught. They grow in their spiritual life much the same way. Your life is the lesson they're learning.

Your unique child may live in a new room—a hospital room—for a while. The following chapter gives hints from those who've made those new rooms home. Even small items brought from home make a huge difference—home to "home."

Through the LORD's mercies we are not consumed,
Because His compassions fail not. They are
new every morning; Great is Your faithfulness.

—Lamentations 3:22-23

5

Making Your Hospital Room Home

It's not easy to feel comfortable in the hospital, but it will be a bit easier if you make your child's hospital room feel homey. As one mom said as she and her CK left the hospital, "I won't miss those four white walls." If you're living with four white walls, or fortunate enough to have a color-decorated children's hospital room, making it home helps your stay. Mostly it helps everyone's mental health. Before you set about the task, make sure you ask about the hospital's rules.

Here are a few ways that your decorations can assist the staff and visitors.

Place a sign on the door to let others know how your CK feels that day. Have your child draw simple faces with a smile or frown and place an arrow with a fastener in the middle, then you can point the arrow to the "feeling" of the hour. You can also add any special messages as they're needed. This is a great tool for facilitating communication. You might also consider placing your child's name in large letters above the head of the bed, like this: "Hi! My name is Julie!" The sign will help everyone coming in the room, and it's nice for your child also.

Decorating Hints

First thing's first. Bring your CK's favorite blankets (quilts), pillow, and stuffed animals from home. The key word is *favorite*. Age doesn't seem to make a difference here. Teens need security blankets also (and so do adults). When you're nestled in the hospital bed, it's comforting to finger the softness of your familiar blanket and snuggle your face into your pillow that smells like home. That's what one CK told us.

Decorating the walls (if it's allowed) can also help. Butterflies? Batman? Boats? What's your child's favorite? Let him decide the theme and give him suggestions on how it can be done (as much as you can do). Also, if you're in and out of the hospital a lot, change the themes. Have your child choose as many of the things displayed as possible.

Themes don't have to be costly. Display your child's art creations, coloring book pictures of the theme, balloons, and toys from home. Also,

Cheer Up!

Your homey hospital room can cheer up the patient, family, friends, and staff. Everyone can use some cheering up!

siblings can color pictures and help with decorations. If you're putting pictures on the walls, avoid cellophane tape, which can pull off paint. You should use poster tack instead, or whatever the hospital suggests.

Time can lose all meaning in the hospital, so put up a schedule for the day. If your child feels well enough, have her check off or use stickers to mark what's been done during the day. This gives her a feeling of accomplishment. The schedule tells your child what to do and when to do it during the day and evening. Your child may find it easier to obey the schedule that tells her what to do than to obey you. And you'll get a break from repeating, "It's time to . . ."

Tips 'n' Tricks

Give the scary IV pole and pump a nickname, then decorate it.

Or you could take photos and make a collage of pictures of staff and other CKs and their families as they come and go.

After a few days (which may seem like weeks or months), both of you will have every detail of the room memorized. A change will help—however slight that may be. Moving chairs, tables, or signs on the walls will be simple. However, if you want to move the bed for more open floor space, ask permission to do so. It may or may not be possible to do that.

Give the scary IV pole and pump a nickname, then decorate it. Tie balloons on it; drape it with colored streamers; hang stuffed animals on it. Camouflage is the key. Others will enjoy seeing the decorated pole and pump maneuvered down the hall by your CK or as it simply decorates the room.

Balloons sent by friends or family are special and they make wonderful decorations. Tie them to the bed or the IV pole;

> ### Humor Helps
>
> You know you've been in the hospital a while when the new nurse asks your child where he lives and he responds, "Here," with a straight face.

you can also attach them to walls. Remember, choose Mylar balloons, not Latex. (Some people are allergic to Latex.) Cards also make wonderful decorations. Hang them on your walls or stick them between the blinds on the window. Save them for later to put in a scrapbook.

Photos make some of the best decorations. Display pictures of your family—including your pets. Put up pictures that show your CK when he or she was healthy. It's great for others to see, and it's wonderful for you to remember and look forward to again. If you think your child is in need of a laugh, ask friends and family to take some pictures making funny faces. When your child is napping, put the funny photos up as a surprise.

Consider hanging a huge blank piece of paper for people to sign their names and write a message. Title it, "My Visitors." You can bless them by writing a positive message across the top for them. Encourage staff to sign it too.

Hints for Passing the Time

Time can move slowly in the hospital, and it may take a little creativity to find enjoyable ways to spend time together—and apart. Here are a few ideas to help you pass the time.

- Enjoy a picnic—on the bed, floor, or tray table—just so you're with the one you love. Be thankful for the food you have, and on special nights order in pizza. "Even Jell-O shared together can be special," a mom said.

- Puzzles and games help keep minds sharp and encourage interaction with others. Bring your favorite games from home, or borrow some from the child life specialist.
- Need a diversion? Watch TV or movies.
- Listen to an iPod or other device. Have headphones handy and put them on for others who need silence—especially if the other person needs a nap.
- If you have memorized every movie you own, you can check out the family resource center for others.
- Take photos or bring some from home and start a scrapbook.
- Touch the world with the Internet. Also, handheld computerized games can be used most anywhere.
- Tack favorite Bible verses and sayings on a poster board to see first thing in the morning—and whenever your child (or you) need a reminder of God's love.
- Make some art. Cut up old calendars with special pictures and make collages. After getting permission, paint windows with washable markers made for glass. Art is a great way to get out feelings. It's good for your child and for the family. You could even try pounding Play-Doh™ or clay for an emotional release. Want a blessing? Make something for somebody else.

- Bring your favorite books from home. Also, check in the family resource center, which probably has shelves of books you've never read.
- Don't forget to create a quiet space. Sometimes a child needs to be alone. Set aside a corner of the room for this. Turn down the lights and add soft music. If your child wants, massage her feet and back with lotion (approved by the nurse).
- Friends can't surround you physically at all times, but try to stay in touch through phone calls, e-mails, and notes. Put up notes received, especially if your child is in isolation.
- Celebrate special occasions or holidays with strings of garland around the room. Choose colors that go with that holiday or your child's favorite colors. Just celebrate. Display your cards on a clothesline tied across the room. If it is Christmas, decorate a small tree. Are you in isolation? Use a ceramic tree. Another suggestion given by a CK, "You can also decorate your IV pole and pump as a tree, which is way cool."
- Give parties for milestones accomplished. Even small steps are steps. Celebrate with family, friends, and staff.

Tips for the Caregiver

When you're the caregiver and you're watching your child cope with such a challenge, it's quite easy to forget yourself. But living at the hospital is tough on you too. Here are some suggestions from caregivers who've lived in the new home. Don't forget to bring the following items from home:

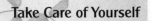

Take Care of Yourself

"Since my child's cancer was the biggie, I ignored my pains—like a toothache, PMS, and meds I was on. But that catches up after a while," a mom said.

Jot notes on things happening to you and what you can do about them.

- Toiletries (necessities!)
- Your meds
- Warm socks or house shoes
- Pictures of family (be sure they have pictures of you and your CK at home)
- Cell phone, Camera (ready for candid shots)
- Water bottles (you can refill them at the sink)
- A special mug for teas and coffee (keep tea bags, hot chocolate, and coffee handy)
- Healthy snacks (to balance out all the others)
- Magazines, books/Kindle, MP3 player, iPod, DVD's
- Journal (for the journey)
- Glasses (and an extra pair if you have one)
- Pillow and a quilt (you need a "blankie" too)
- Thank you notes to slip to others (pray to see their needs through God's eyes)
- Your own unique things to make the room feel homier for you
- List of names, phone numbers, and e-mail addresses to keep in touch with everyone
- List of who is doing what and who you need to thank

- Calendars, pencils, pens, and stickers (you could use some smiley-face stickers too)
- Your Bible and a devotional book (a suggested list of these books are in the Bibliography and Resource Three). Put Bible verses and quotes on cards to set out or stick on the mirror (you never know when you might need the encouragement).

Having everything you need on hand in the hospital room will make you more comfortable and give you some control. Keep your calendar/journal and pen handy as you schedule things and keep track of your family at home. Contact information for family and friends is invaluable. It's easy to forget even familiar phone numbers when you're stressed and running on empty.

Here are a few more suggestions for you, the caregiver, to help life run as smoothly as possible during a bumpy time.

- Leave recipes and helpful hints for Mr. Mom at home—or whoever is there. Keep a list of any allergies anyone has. Mark them in red!
- Leave notes at home for your family—from you and your CK. Write short notes of encouragement to the CK's siblings. Good luck in your game tonight! Hope your math test goes well! Thanks for cleaning

the bathroom! Whatever it might be, there are still things going on in their lives.

- Keep all papers together, if possible. Use a BIG notebook with dividers or a box with dividers. This big notebook is separate from the HUGE notebook you may have received from the staff when your CK was first admitted.
- Get baskets or containers to hold many of the items you and your child need at the hospital (for quick and easy transport from home to hospital . . . to home . . .)

Tips 'n' Tricks

Find "homes" for the many new papers and items on this new journey. To save precious time and energy, put things back where they belong—each time—in their place. An accordion file or color-coded files for each category is helpful with all the paperwork. Also, have someone help you organize the papers and assist you if needed. Sometimes you need that "second brain" to think through situations.

The demanding cancer journey requires stamina. As you make the hospital environment more pleasant, you nurture your child and yourself. Both of you need extra strength to cope with overwhelming tests and treatments. In the next chapter we'll look at some tips to help you through those times. Hang in there. You'll make it!

There is something about keeping him (God) divine that keeps him distant, packaged, predictable. But don't do it. For heaven's sake, don't. Let him be as human as he intended to be. Let him into the mire and muck of our world. For only if we let him in can he pull us out.

—Max Lucado

6

Forewarned Is Forearmed

Part of the mire and muck of this journey may include chemotherapy and radiation. Forewarned *is* forearmed as fellow travelers give the following helpful hints. Also, ask your health professionals about new information and ways to deal with these side effects.

K is for Kemo

As you walk down the halls of children's hospitals, splashes of bright colors cover the walls and pull you into their world. In one hospital I visited, teens painted the alphabet, and each letter had an accompanying picture that dealt with cancer. Halfway down the hall hung this sign: K is for Kemo.

So what about chemotherapy? And mainly, what about the side effects? The following are suggestions from CKs and their families who've dealt with "kemo." We'll list the various side effects and some suggestions for ways to handle the worst of it. Of course, you'll find out what works best for your child. Also, physicians, nurses, and other patients will have helpful suggestions for you.

- **Losing hair.** One young patient suggested, "Cut it really short soon. It falls out in clumps, and that's awful. My mom and dad made a big deal about it—sort of like a party. And tell the kids, it will grow back." Some boys don't take it as hard as girls and are disappointed when their hair grows back and it looks different. Some want it shaved again!
- **Nausea.** Your child may say, "I'm getting the throw-up medicine again." You should carry a bucket, wipes, extra towels, and mouthwash at all times. Stash them in the car, especially for your drive home after the chemo treatment. Actually, keep them everywhere your CK may be. Anything can set off the nausea, so ask the nurse for anti-nausea drugs before it hits. Keep a record of when it hits, what brings it on, and which meds work.
- **Fatigue.** It will hit, so plan ahead. Don't let your CK overdo it, but do things that help release endorphins (see Chapter Seven), such as laughing, walking, and playing games. "You don't think that fatigue is a big deal? Think about the most exhausting day you've ever had, or the worst flu, and times it by ten," a

grandmother said, who'd survived chemo herself.

- **Sores in the mouth and throat.** Slowly suck on red popsicles, not citrus-flavored ones, which have too much acid. Suck on candy like Jolly Ranchers® or whatever candies work for you. Here's a suggestion from Rochelle, a young doctor who personally battled cancer

> **Save Your Energy**
>
> Keep your eye on the gas gauge. Fill up when you're approaching a quarter of a tank. Don't push it to the "E." You never know when you'll need to make a trip to the ER, especially in the middle of the night.

and dealt with chemo as a patient: "Chemo causes a wretched taste in your mouth, but I learned a secret remedy. Suck on Sour Patch Kids candy (sour lemon drops weren't sour enough) before you eat a meal. It forces this huge surge of the wretched taste and then you can rinse your mouth out and manage most, if not all, of a meal before the taste comes back."

- **Counts go down.** Beware who your child is around, because lowered white blood cells can't do their job and the CK is vulnerable to infectious diseases. For a while, this is drive-thru McDonald's time, not inside playground time.
- **Stay out of direct sunlight.** It may seem overprotective, but it's not. Slap on sunblock even if it's a cold or cloudy day. Your CK is more susceptible to sunburns.

- **Parents' unexpected feelings.** A mom said, "As bad as the side effects are, you still feel like something's being done. When you're in remission, you feel strangely lost. You don't have a place to go on certain days, and realize that it is now up to you. That can be a scary and lonely feeling. I didn't expect that." Parents, please ask for help when your child is on chemo, and ask for help when he's not on chemo. The staff is only a phone call away.

'Roid Rage

"How bad can it be? I had a steroid shot when my shoulder went out," a dad said. "I did have some appetite gain, slept a little less, but, wow, what energy I had. So, it really wasn't that bad."

One shot? Now multiply that to a near toxic megadose. That's a steroid pulse given to a CK to kill the aggressive cancer cells. It's a life-saving treatment. As one mom said, "You should describe the side effects first—no wait, don't. No one would sign the consent form. But it helps save these precious lives."

Forewarned is forearmed. Like "kemo," these side effects too shall pass. Let's take a quick look at what to expect when your CK receives steroids.

> ### Let's Pray about Chemo
>
> Dear Lord,
>
> Please help the chemo to attack the bad and bypass the good cells. Thank you for the treatments we have in this country. Many countries don't have treatment, hospitals, or care for their children at all. Even through the treatments are tough, we are so grateful for them. Amen.

- **Weight gain**. Keep five sizes of clothes handy (before, during, during, during, and after)
- **Appearance**. Moon-shaped face and belly
- **Appetite**. Eating everything in sight and craving whatever isn't in sight (cravings may change frequently)· Mood swings that make extreme PMS seem normal
- **Energy**. Energy swings will be common

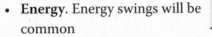

Let's Pray about Steroids

Dear God,

Please walk us through these steroid days. I know I'll need more patience—lots more patience and understanding. I thank you for your promises to always be with us. Amen.

Steroids can be a rough patch on the treatment road. As one parent said, "One of the hardest things can be taking your seemingly well child and making him sick again, but that's part of the journey." Another mom shared, "I go from my four-year-old not being able to run, or even walk, to steroid-induced frenzies. I'd give anything for a regular running event. Maybe one of these days."

Of course, the side effects are most difficult for the kids themselves. One teen CK said, "My two-year-old brother won't come near me and play right now. I look so different, and he's not sure what's going on. I don't feel like a sister anymore." A child life specialist can help patient and siblings to cope not just with the diagnosis but with the treatments and their side effects.

Steroid treatment can be quite draining. You and your CK should get as much sleep as possible to replenish what the steroids zap (easier said than done unless you're on the verge of collapse). Spending some time simply relaxing is beneficial as well. Of course, it's hard to truly relax when you're feeling worried. Even though worry is futile and depletes our strength, it's hard to let go of it. Ask God to help you let it go.

Caregiver, you're riding the waves of side effects as they slam on the shoreline boulders. Then you catch your breath as the waves recede and you float on the white foam. In the distance, you spot the next breaker building. But for the present minutes, hours, or days, you rest in the calm. Let God join you in the calm and in the chaos. He's been in both.

Focus not just on the unfairness and problems of life, but also on all that does turn out well. Review the good things of the past, and don't forget in the darkness what you've learned in the light.

—Phillip Yancey

7

Caring for the Caregiver

With a cancer diagnosis comes loss of control, fears for the future, lack of privacy, ravaged routines, and financial worries—and those are just the obvious onslaughts. In the midst of this, who takes care of the caregiver? Only the caregiver can add this responsibility to the never-ending list, but they rarely do. Why don't caregivers take care of themselves? Here are some typical responses:

- "But I'm not the sick one. I feel guilty even thinking about my needs."
- "I hardly have the energy to take care of my CK, much less myself."
- "My brain is foggy all the time, so I just wander from one decision to the next."

These answers all sound valid, but what's the bottom line? If the caregiver goes down the tube, the rest of the family will too. It's hard to recognize this problem when you're in the midst of a crisis, but it's real, and moms are often the ones who fall prey to it. We've heard many dads say, "She thinks she's the only one who can do it right." And that is understandable, but what is the outcome? Compassion fatigue.

Compassion, of course, is a good thing, but compassion fatigue isn't good for anyone. You care deeply about your child, but you can care too much.

"Care too much? You can't care too much," one mom said. "I just can't leave my child's side—ever. I'm getting sleep; fifteen minutes at a time adds up. Okay, so I'm also snacking, but I'm really not hungry. You don't understand. I have to be here 24/7, and I'm sorry, but no one else can do this. This is my whole life."

But what is the result? Fatigue. Compassion fatigue drains precious energy, and it is not a respecter of persons. It's an equal opportunity problem that can attack parents, family, doctors, nurses—all the people in your child's life. Caring and sympathy are good things, just counterproductive when taken to the extreme.

To relieve compassion fatigue and provide yourself with a bit of caretaking, do your best to connect with yourself, with others, and with God on a regular basis. These connections are vital to give you strength to continue the journey. They act like a shot of endorphins and they'll help you take better care of your CK.

This chapter looks at ways to make these connections within the framework of your overwhelmed, fatigued life.

Connecting With Self

One of the most important ways to connect with yourself is to plan ahead with your calendar and notebook/journal. Your mind is crammed with schedules, tests, protocols, when and where siblings need to be, who is dropping off food for your family tonight (always a good thing), and the fact that your house is a wreck (which feels like a bad thing). In the middle of juggling all those thoughts in your head, you might think, "Did I call Susan back yesterday?" On it goes.

Now, slow down, and take a deep breath. Grab your pen, and write everything that you need to do. If you're still feeling overwhelmed, prioritize the list. Rank the tasks in the order of importance to be done. Read it every night and every morning, and check off what you've accomplished. Prioritize what needs to be done for the next day.

The notebook may become your new best friend. It will tell you what to do, and you won't waste precious energy trying to remember whatever you were supposed to remember. Keep the notebook with you, and several pens and pencils with it. Pens and pencils mysteriously disappear when you need them, so plan ahead. For a dollar you can get a pack of eight pens at most stores.

Still overwhelmed by the uncontrollable situation? Pray the words written by Reinhold Neibuhr, "God, grant me the serenity to accept the things I cannot change, courage to change the things I can, and wisdom to know the difference."

Forgetfulness Is Okay

"But I'm sure I won't forget." Yes, you will. It's to be expected.

Ability

List the things you can change, and then tackle the list. Put the rest on the back burner.

Stress sends out a barrage of negative messengers (adrenaline and cortisol in particular) in the brain, throwing us into fight-or-flight mode. We may overly react in anger or run away from the problem. To combat stress, we have to choose to jumpstart the positive messengers—endorphins. Endorphin is a substance in the brain that attaches to the same cell receptors that morphine does. It abolishes the sensation of pain. The brain doesn't know if the person is really happy, it just responds to the happy messengers. Result? We feel better.

Endorphins are needed in all phases of life to help our physical and emotional states. They also boost the immune system. Fortunately, we can add some activities into our daily routine (or lack thereof) to release those precious endorphins. Let's look at ways to do that.

Laughter!

"I don't think I'll ever be able to laugh again," a mom said. Then another mom added, "One day I caught myself laughing at something on TV and I felt guilty. My kids were relieved to hear me laugh, and it opened a discussion about our new normal, which had little laughter. We all seemed to need permission to laugh."

Laughter (inside jogging) oxygenates your entire body, which is desperately needed during stressful times. Is your blood pressure up? Depression and tension setting in? Having trouble digesting your food? Try a dose of laughter!

Sometimes we'd like someone else to initiate our laughter. We'd like to have someone tickle us, or tell a joke—then we'd totally laugh our heads off, and not think of anything but laughing and gasping for air! But that's probably not going to happen, so you'll need to take matters into your own hands.

Now, what's funny to you? Watch a slapstick movie, read a humorous book, or listen to a ridiculous CD. Find a five-year-old and have them tell you a knock-knock joke—then watch them bend over with laughter. It's contagious.

Check out the Never-Ending Squirrel Tale website and click, "You know you're the parent of a kid with cancer when. . . ." Here are a few of the hundreds listed by parents. You know you're the parent of a kid with cancer when . . .

- You start teaching your daughter the parts of her body, and you point to her chest and she says that's her port.
- Medical students ask to borrow your notes.
- Your toddler refuses to sit on Santa's lap because he's too germy from all the other kids.

Only families of CKs relate to this list and get it. As you read the list on the website, not only will you laugh, you'll remember you're not alone.

Sleep

Sleep is another powerful way to release endorphins. To refurbish your body, you need six to eight hours of sleep. REM sleep (rapid eye movement) occurs in cycles, and especially during the last few hours when you're dreaming. The early hours give rest for the body, but the later hours renew and rebuild it. This

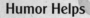

Humor Helps

You can sleep anywhere, and anything that reclines more than fifteen degrees looks "comfy."

recommendation may seem impossible, knowing how hard it is to get the sleep needed, but it is important.

One CK's dad said, "It seems weird. You're so tired, you'd think you'd fall asleep and stay asleep. But being that exhausted, you can't fall asleep, and then you toss and turn. Or, if you do fall asleep, you wake up in the middle of the night, your mind races, and you can't go back to sleep. It's really strange."

Whether you're in the hospital room, at home, staying in the Ronald McDonald house, or wherever you're trying to rest, attempt to get eight hours of sleep—even if it's interrupted. You also may need to switch off occasionally with a family member or friend and have them spend the night with your child. Results? You have a fresh viewpoint in the morning as your body, mind, and emotions are renewed. You need that REM sleep for the long haul.

How do you feel when you cuddle your sleeping child? You want them comfortable and serene, and you'll do whatever it takes to have that happen. That's how God feels when he watches any of his children sleep. He wants you comfortable and serene—safe in his arms.

If you (or your CK) is sleeping fitfully these days, LaDonna Meinders, author of *Angel Hugs for Cancer Patients*, shares this idea in her book. Sheets and pillowcases wad into wrinkles during fitful sleep. Turning the pillow over to the cool side relieves the heat and moisture from your face. After flipping the pillow, nestle in, and thank God for his care.

Eight hours (even interrupted) is ideal, but some nights you'll get little or no sleep and then fall asleep in the middle of the day. Try to schedule a power nap between various visitors and staff coming and going. Dim the lights and curl up with your blankie. Set a quiet alarm for fifteen to thirty minutes. You'll probably wake up groggy, but that goes away and you'll have a surge of energy to carry you through the evening.

Exercise

Exercise is another way to release endorphins. You may be thinking, "Oh yeah, when is that supposed to happen?" Time is indeed a problem, but we're not talking about a full workout here.

Walk laps up and down the hospital hall, take the stairs to the cafeteria, or pump iron (two eight-ounce cans of food will do). It doesn't take much because anything helps. Ten minutes of walking gets your blood flowing. It needs the help. Ten minutes three times a day is fantastic.

The family room on your floor may have a treadmill. Take advantage of it. If you're at home and your children are old enough to leave for a few minutes, walk up and down your block. If they're not old enough, then walk in your house and turn up your favorite "walking" music. If you have a treadmill at home, that's even better exercise to keep the blood flowing. Also do exercises while sitting in your chair, stretching your arms, leaning your head side to side, extending your legs.

There's an added benefit while you're in the hospital: walking requires leaving the room. This may be very difficult for mom, but it's needed. Pace

> **The Journey**
> Pace yourself. This journey is a marathon, not a short run.

yourself. Again, this journey is a marathon, not a short run. By taking even ten minutes to exercise, you aren't just caring for yourself—you're doing the best thing for everyone else too.

Sunshine

Open those blinds and turn on lots of lamps. Light increases your level of serotonin, a hormone that helps elevate your mood and decrease fatigue. On this journey, you definitely want some serotonin to give you more energy and courage to face the day.

However, the amount of light your child can tolerate depends on your CK's condition, so check with the nurse first.

Deep Breaths

Bring oxygen deep down into your lungs through your nose, count to five, and then breathe out through your mouth. As you breathe out you release toxins from your body. Repeat ten times, three times a day.

This clears your brain, burns calories, and relaxes the body. It's free. What more can you ask?

> **God's Promise**
>
> You will keep him in perfect peace, *Whose* mind *is* stayed *on You*, Because he trusts in You.
> —Isaiah 26:3

Also, drink lots of water. "Drink water? But it doesn't have caffeine!"

As stress bombards your body, toxins (poisons) are building. Deep breaths release toxins from your body and water flushes them out. (Yes, that means frequenting the bathroom.) Try to get eight ounces, six times a day. Keep filling that water bottle!

Food

Food also has a powerful effect on the way we feel, and stress can have a profound impact on the way we eat. "I'm just not hungry," one mom said. And her friend replied, "I just eat all the time."

Where's the balance?

"At the family support group, we always brought food," Hedy said. "Guess what everyone brought? Pizza! It was fast, easy, comfort food. Just what you need as you sit by the hour in the hospital room—oh, and cookies too. You talk about a vicious cycle. You're exhausted, then you overdose on caffeine and sugar to keep you awake at night to check on things. When you come down off the caffeine and sugar you get depressed, so you hit those foods and drinks again. Smart, huh?

"Well, we know it's a crutch, but those long hours, either in the hospital or at home—it just happens. I'd tell parents to try to watch what and when they're eating. You don't even realize it until you look at all the empty cans, Styrofoam containers, and cookie wrappers."

If you keep a journal, take notes not only of what your CK is eating and drinking, but you too. Your body has got to be the best it can be for everyone's sake.

> **Tips 'n' Tricks**
>
> Keep crunchy fruit, vegetables, and healthy snacks handy.
>
> If there is a refrigerator on the floor for families to use, store your food in baggies and label them with your name.
>
> Also, stock up on multivitamins.

Connecting With Others

"I never thought I'd ever shut people out of my life, but as I've become wearier, that's what I've done," said a mom. "I know others really care, but I don't have the strength at times to talk. How can I explain things over and over and over . . ."

Internet and E-Mail

It can be overwhelming to try to stay connected to all your loved ones and all the people who care about your child. Check into the websites CaringBridge (www.caringbridge. com) or CarePages (www.carepages.com) for free, personal, easy-to-create web pages that help you connect with friends and family (see Resource Four). You can create a page for your child and post regular updates. This will allow friends and family to stay connected to your family at a time when you may have little time for phone calls. You may want to keep the site updated yourself, but there may be days (or nights) when you can't. You may also choose to have someone else keep up the site for you.

However, many parents find when they e-mail others or post to a personal website, it is an outlet for their emotions—a catharsis. And of course, it's a blessing to read the e-mails or posts made in response. Those prayers and encouraging words will uplift you and your child. Communication goes both ways.

Connect Online

You might want to add a note like this one to your CarePage or CaringBridge site: "Your messages on our CarePage encourage our hearts. But whether you leave a message or not, thanks for keeping up with us and for the prayers. Only heaven will reveal the silent prayer warriors!"

Ask for Help

Asking for help does a lot to forge connections with family and friends. No one can read your mind. You'll have needs your family and friends have never thought about unless they've been on this journey. Even if they have, all situations are different. If you've had to be "the strong one," it will be difficult to ask for help. Remember, this isn't about you; this is about quality time for your CK—which is enhanced if you've asked for help.

CarePages Help

One mom wrote,

"Reading other people's CarePages and what they've been through with BMTs (bone marrow transplants) helps me know what's coming and what to do."

When friends say, "How can I help?" tell them. Make a list with specifics—from cleaning your house, bringing meals, and watching the siblings to simply coming and sitting with you to talk—and to let you catch a quick shower. "Showers have never felt so good," most moms say.

In Person

Although there's great value in connecting with others, it can also be difficult to do so. You're living a reality most people will never experience. When bombarded with too many inquiries about how you're doing, just muster a slight smile and say, "We're exhausted, but thank you for asking." You'll never have the time or ability to completely explain your new life to them.

If you're a more introverted Blue or Green personality, dealing with other people wears you out. To be refilled you need your quiet space and time. To set your boundaries with others, rehearse what you will say (remembering to thank them for their thoughtfulness). Have an outgoing Yellow family member or friend be the contact person for you most of the time. It will give you the space you need to regroup and will use your Yellow friend's strength, which will bring her joy interacting with others.

Do you want to be kept in the loop with friends? You've probably forgotten there is a loop—the outside world, your former life before cancer. Have friends keep you up on what's going on, but beware. When they tell you about the outside world, they'll talk about their lives—their lives with healthy children, no clinics, no pain.

You may end up feeling like this mom: "I want to hear, I really do. But I get jealous when I think what their kids can do and mine can't."

Pray for an open heart to listen to others. Those parents don't know what to say to you; you be their guide. You need them, and they need to hear from you. While it's important to maintain your connections with those in the outside world, it's also valuable to reach out to those inside your new world. You need those other foggy-brained families wandering around the hospital, in the clinics, and at support groups and camps.

You may think, "But I've only begun this journey; some have been on it a long time." Everyone has something to add to the other's journey. Remember, you're their best resource and know how they feel as few others do.

Connecting With God

It's easy to see that you can connect inwardly with yourself and horizontally with others. But you can also connect vertically with God. The following pages shed more light on this dark journey as you connect with him through the Bible (his Word to you), prayer (talking and listening to him), journaling (seeing how He's working in your life), music, and appreciating his creation. God constantly reaches out to you. Each of us is uniquely touched by him.

We've talked about Gary Chapman's book, *The Five Love Languages*, which discusses the way humans interact and love one another. To understand connecting with God more fully, read Chapman's book *The Five Love Languages of God*. As 1 John 4:19 says, "We love [God] because He first loved us."

Humor Helps

You know you're a mother of a cancer kid when you can get up every hour to hit the beeping IV button, empty puke buckets every other hour, and still call it a good night's sleep.

Talk and Listen to Him

You may feel as if your life has been struck by continuous waves as you lie weary on the beach. But you're not alone. God the Father is always there ready to help. Dr. Brand experienced God in the midst of overwhelming situations. He gave this analogy in his book, *In His Image*: many ships navigate using radar equipment and landmarks. However, before the days of radar, when sailors were surrounded by open sea (no landmarks), they depended entirely on sextants, two tubes joined at a hinge.

All day they watched the sea, all night, the stars. To get a precise reading of where they were, they needed a clear sighting of both a certain star and the only fixed point, the horizon, to determine an angle. Only two times of day, dawn and dusk, offered such conditions, bringing heaven and earth together.

"It captures the concept of planting my feet firmly on earth while sighting along a line of spiritual direction. I need a time of day to orient myself, to bring heaven and earth together. In the midst of the clamor and tumult of this material world, I must find a place of quietness to listen to the still, small voice for guidance of my life."

He further said,

"To survive, I must pause to breathe in the power of the living God and consciously direct my mind to Him."

Dr. Brand devoted his life to lepers in India and other third world countries. His life overflowed with "clamor and tumult" on earth, but he drew his strength from heaven.

A CK's mom in Baltimore said, "I began strong with praying, but over time I was so worn down that I prayed less and I felt guilty. But that's when the Holy Spirit took over and I knew He prayed on my behalf."

As Romans 8:26 says, "Likewise the Spirit also helps in our weaknesses. For we do not know what we should pray for as we ought, but the Spirit Himself makes intercession for us with groanings which cannot be uttered." When you feel like you don't even have a prayer left, remember that the Holy Spirit is our translator to God our Father—with our spoken and unspoken prayers.

Read His Word

"E-mails are getting too impersonal. I need to handwrite a letter to my daughter," reflected a mom:

"My precious child, I just wanted you to know how much I love you, and am proud of you. Remember that no matter what, I am always here to help. . . . [The letter continued flowing with words of encouragement.]

—Love, Mom

Mom folded the letter, slipped it into the envelope, and mailed it.

Two days passed, the daughter sorted through her mail, and the handwritten envelope brought a smile. "That was nice of Mom to write me," then she tossed it unopened on the coffee table and mumbled, "I'll read it later when I have time."

The next day her mom dropped by, and after hugs, the phone rang.

"I'll be right back," the daughter said, and then she left the room. Mom settled on the sofa and noticed the opened letters, bills, and magazines strewn on the coffee table. Sticking out underneath the stack, she saw her letter, unopened. Entering the room, her daughter caught her mom's disappointed glance, and quickly said, "I haven't had time to read it, but I will."

Her unspoken words said, "I really don't care very much." She missed the blessing.

"How rude," I thought, reading the story. Then I looked at my coffee table littered with *opened* mail, bills, and magazines, which all covered my Bible plopped down on Sunday after church. My quick response, "I haven't had time to read it, but I will." My unspoken words said, "I really don't care very much."

> ### Make Some Time
> We make time for what's important in our lives. Get to know God personally by reading his letter to you—then work his words into your life.

My Heavenly Father wants me to know how much he cares; He has plans and protection for me. And yes, without reading his heart in words, I miss the blessing.

Journal

Whether writing by hand or using a computer, it's amazing to keep track of God's work in your life, especially on this journey. If you don't have a journal, a simple pad of paper will do. Be honest in your feelings. God is not offended—or surprised. Is the new normal still smothering you? Pick the petals off a daisy, but change the words: "he loves me, he loves me, he loves me. . . ."

Yes, he does. You'll realize this more and more as you count your blessings. Count them first thing in the morning as you struggle out of bed and the last thing at night as you collapse into it. Count them while you sit on the sofa or scrunch close to your child in the hospital's single bed. Try it during the night as you smack the beeping IV button. You do have blessings, but probably can't remember them because your mind is crammed with the new normal. Take time to think about it, and write them down when you have a chance.

If you're thinking, "Blessings? What blessings?" we have some suggestions from fellow travelers.

- "I can see with both eyes. It's that simple; something I took for granted, then I had a problem with my eye and realized how important that was."
- "Being able to get this kind of special care and treatment for my child. In my home country, he would have died."

- "Strangers, who smile at me in the elevator even when I'm standing there in my grubby clothes and I haven't put on makeup."
- "Cafeteria food. Even though I'm sick of eating the same things, it is downstairs."
- "Pinks of sunrise. I've seen lots of them, and they bring hope for a new day after a long dark night. They're especially beautiful as a backdrop for black silhouetted trees."
- "Knowing I can count on others to pray for us. They really care."

Start your own "Thanks-giving" list. Read it over every morning as you wake. God will plant new patterns of thinking (thanksgiving) in your brain. After all, he's your Spiritual Caregiver who never becomes weary of giving care.

Communicate Through Music

Music stirs our heartstrings, and surfaces our emotions. Open a Bible to the middle. There you'll find King David's songs from his heart—the Psalms. They're still touching hearts today—our hearts and the heart of God. Long ago, David said, "The LORD *is* my strength and my shield; My heart trusted in Him, and I am helped; Therefore my heart greatly rejoices, And with my song I will praise Him" (Ps. 28:7).

Words from the hymn "Count Your Blessings," written in 1897, still speak to strugglers today:

Praise & Thanksgiving

Praise focuses on who God is, while thanksgiving focuses on what God does.

107

When upon life's billows you are tempest tossed.
When you are discouraged, thinking all is lost.
Count your many blessings name them one by one.
And it will surprise you what the Lord has done.

Blessings continue each day—just keep your eyes on him. When you look, you will be surprised what the Lord has done.

Tunes and beats change from one generation to the next, but they still connect people to God. Pastor Dave Slagle shared this story in a sermon: "Driving down the road, radio blaring, the three of us sang with the praise music. In the back seat, three-year-old Jack was totally into 'Holy, holy, Lord of heaven and earth!'

"As we pulled up to the house, I switched off the radio, but Jack continued singing. This time we heard his words. 'Hode me, hode me, Lord of heaben and earth!' The words were wrong, but the message was right.

"God wants us to come as trusting children, throwing our arms up to him, and saying, 'Hode me.' He's been waiting to do just that."

Sometimes it's easiest to ask God for help by using the words to a song. Don't hesitate to do that.

Appreciate His Creation

Reality

"The Bible is more real than the book you are holding in your hands."

—Brennan Manning

Ever notice how most of the world is either blue or green? Blue water covers most of our globe, blue skies arch from horizon to horizon, and green vegetation sprouts in trees and grasses. Why so much blue and green? They're calm, cool colors. God knew we would need a majority of calm colors in our hectic lives with occasional splashes of bright reds, yellows, and other colors in the spectrum.

"The heavens declare the glory of God; And the firmament shows His handiwork," Psalm 19:1 says.

Don't miss a day appreciating his handiwork. Early morning or evening, step outside or peek through a window at the rising or setting of the sun, as pinkish-orange rays begin or end a day in your life.

Familiarity creeps in as the majesty of our created world becomes humdrum. We take it for granted because we see it every day. Ask God for a fresh viewpoint, then gaze at whatever creation is nearby.

Look closely at any flower—the colors in any flower always blend. The hues compliment each other and never clash. Another one of the Creator's coincidences.

What are some scenes that bring peace to your heart? Endless beaches with tufts of wild grass blown by salty sprays of seawater? Majestic mountain ranges, carved by deep valleys? Sunshine backlighting long-needle pines or icicles drooping them to the ground?

Frame a picture copied off the Internet, cut from a magazine, or from a trip you enjoyed. Choose somewhere to place a small bowl of shells or rocks collected from a special place. Have live plants nearby. This will depend on your CK's condition—always check with the nurses first when dealing with live plants and flowers. Items that display the beauty of the earth remind us of the Creator of that beauty.

Over two thousand years ago, Jesus spoke to crowds on a hillside. He told them not to worry, because they couldn't add a single hour to their life. Then he added not to even worry about clothes. ". . . Consider the lilies of the field, how they grow: they neither toil nor spin; and yet I say to you that even Solomon in all his glory was not arrayed like one of these" (Matt. 6:28-29).

He is the Creator of everything created. Connect with him.

Now connect with family as you fly with your flock in the next chapter. Everyone in your flock needs encouragement for the long flight as their weary wings flap, buffeted by storm clouds.

We cannot change our past . . . we cannot change the fact that people act in a certain way. We cannot change the inevitable. The only thing we can do is play on the one string we have, and that is our attitude. I am convinced that life is 10 percent what happens to me and 90 percent how I react to it.

—Charles Swindoll

Family Flocks

Let's consider some lessons from the wobbly V. You hear them before you see them. Suddenly, they swoosh overhead, the wobbly V of Canada geese gliding across the horizon, honking encouragement to one another for their extensive journey.

Cancer families endure long journeys too, and desperately need encouragement. Some of that encouragement comes packaged in humor.

"You know how geese always fly in a V formation, but do you know why one line of the V is always longer than the other? Give up? Because there are more birds in the longer one! Ha! Thought you'd like that. Get better soon." This comment was found on a CarePage. It was written from a teacher to her former student with cancer.

Soaring

When you hear the soothing cadence of honking—look up. A flock is soaring.

Surprisingly perhaps, we can learn from flocks of flying geese. Let these lessons strengthen your weary wings.

In a flock of geese flying in V formation, the lead goose rotates back in the formation when it grows tired. Are you the lead goose? Are you the main caregiver on the cancer journey? If so, you may feel you can never rotate back and must take the lead, 24/7. Besides, what would others think if you weren't there all the time?

The fact is, dear lead goose, you *are* on an extremely long journey. Take the opportunity to rotate back at times. Others will need you for the extensive journey.

Canada geese work together as they migrate. Each bird in the V flaps its wings, creating an uplift for the following bird, thereby traveling seventy-one percent further than if each bird flew on its own, as all head in the same direction. Cancer families, too, need to uplift each other for their extensive journey. And the flock needs to fly in the same direction. There are a number of ways to make that happen. Your CK doesn't need to hear conflicting advice.

For example, Mom may say, "He needs more rest."

Dad may respond, "No, he needs to get out of that bed."

Do your best to communicate your ideas and listen to others' opinions. If you do disagree about strategies for your CK, discuss the disagreement in private.

Each goose's special cadence "Honk!" inspires courage. "Keep on going!" However, if a goose has to drop out of formation, another goose (or two) drops out and flies alongside him. If he lands to recoup, the other two stay with him until they can all rejoin the flock.

In the same way, each family member inspires courage with special words and actions to "Keep on going!" However, there may be times when a family member needs to drop out of formation with the flock. This may be due to health, emotional overload, or other hindering circumstances. Others (immediate or extended family) need to be aware and come alongside until that member is able to join the flock again. Understandably, most of the family's attention is directed toward the CK—so keep your eyes open for others who may need help.

In the darkness, geese continue to communicate by honking, so no goose gets lost.

By effective communication, talking and listening to each other, no one in the family gets lost in the darkness, and all stay connected. Your family may have had great coping skills in the past; if so, those skills will probably help you. However, this is an entirely new journey. Unlike geese that follow the same migration path year after year, you and your flock have not traveled this way before. Individuals' thoughts on issues may change daily—even hourly—so take time each day to share those feelings. Holding them in is counterproductive, but remember to share them in love.

In your flock, a united front may be divided over finances, rules for siblings at home, even parents' faith. "I know God will heal him," a father may say about his son. That rings hollow to the spouse who chides, "This is the real world of cancer we're dealing with." Be patient and tolerant of your differences. Again, they make sense to the other person.

Another part of your life that needs attention is your sexual relationship. "But I feel guilty seeking pleasure in the midst of all this," a mom said. "Besides, I'm too exhausted." A dad added, "And I'm worn down worrying about finances. I never even have time to shave. I look perpetually stubbly."

Plan ahead and take the time needed to stay close and reassured of each other's love.

Generations Fly Alongside

"I don't know what I would have done without my mother," said the young woman holding her toddler. "I know it's killing her watching all this, but she's been a rock."

You may or may not have help from your parents. If you do, you may not view some things they say and do as a help.

How do grandparents come alongside without taking over? It isn't easy. They not only worry about their grandchild, but also their child—two generations of worrying you'd call it. Their emotional tanks have emptied also.

Many emotional and interpersonal issues come to the surface on this journey. As the generations try to work together, things can get tough. Some parents have voiced these feelings:

> **God's Promise**
>
> Children's children *are* the crown of old men, And the glory of children *is* their father.
>
> —Proverbs 17:6

- "I'm glad Mom and Dad are here, but . . . "
- "They make me feel inadequate, second-guessing my decisions."
- "They sigh all the time—especially around their grandson."

(Review the Blue personality who feel others' pain deeply.)

- "They instruct the nurses and anyone else who walks in the room on how they should do their job." (Review Red personality who makes sure everything is done right.)

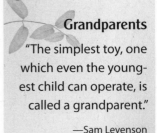

Grandparents

"The simplest toy, one which even the youngest child can operate, is called a grandparent."

—Sam Levenson

- "I guess the bottom line is that all the old bad things (memories) rise to the top, and I can't deal with those and the new bad things."

If any of these thoughts ring true, now is the time to confront lovingly. You may be surprised at unspoken thoughts lodged in your parents' minds as everyone continues reeling. Plan ahead on what to say, where to say it, and, most importantly, how to say it.

What to say? Here are a few brief ideas:

- "Mom and Dad, thanks so much for your support. We're really going to need it for the long haul. We need a time to sit and talk with you out of hearing range of the children, because we're all running on empty emotionally, and we need to have a game plan."
- "(Child's name) needs all of us to be on the same page dealing with his medical care. He needs us to be as positive as possible because he can read our body language. Smiles are necessary, and we have to watch the sighing. Actually, this is true for all our children. We're all in this together, and we may need

to touch base like this each day for a while."

Where do you say it? Away from the children. How do you say it? Respectfully.

The Rest of the Flock

Probably many of your child's aunts, uncles, and cousins are chiming in, "We're here for you." Whether they're near or far, keep them in the loop, through email and calls. One person may be the point person to contact the others.

Whoever is in your flock, refer to the You-niquely Made Personality Study in Resource One for a refresher on your gene pool. Remember, Reds will direct family and staff, Blues will sigh and straighten the room (let them), Yellows will talk constantly to other families and staff (but probably won't remember their names), and Greens will sit for hours lending a listening ear to anyone who needs it. Appreciate each member of your flock.

Flying Through the Holidays

All the holidays can be difficult in the new normal. Roller-coaster emotions soar and dive as families remember previous holidays, struggle through the current one, and anticipate the next ones. Emotions are stretched to the limit. Especially around the holidays, you may find yourself feeling like this mom: "One day we feel blessed, and the next blasted. I'm praying for a balance. Only God can give that, because we can't ourselves."

New Year's

The new normal brings a different perspective on New Year's resolutions. Losing a few pounds or giving up a bad habit pale in comparison to your new life. Looking at January of the new year, you're struck with the preciousness of life, health (in whatever condition that may be), and hopefulness for the future. January 1 pushes you forward.

Plan ahead. Flip the calendar to the upcoming months and write something special to do for someone once a month or more frequently if you can. It may be very small in your sight, but not in God's. Pray for his guidance through each of the 365 days.

Easter

"I knew Thanksgiving and Christmas were going to be difficult in the hospital, but I never thought about Easter. It hit hard," a mom said.

Feeling hopeless? Take a look back at the first Easter—actually, three days before Easter. Good Friday we now call it. Jesus died on a bloody cross and all hope was gone, even for Jesus' family and followers.

Next came Saturday—and God didn't show up. It looked like Satan had won the victory and Jesus was silenced for good.

Then early on the third day after his death, as grieving women came to his tomb, they found the huge stone that covered the doorway rolled away. The tomb was empty!

Over the next forty days, more than five hundred people saw and talked with the resurrected Jesus before he ascended back to Heaven. He won the victory over death, and from there we have hope—hope in life, and hope in death. The Resurrection.

God had been working in the darkness! And God still works in the darkness of our lives.

Read his story in chapters 17-21 in the book of John.

Mother's Day!

One CK's mom said, "I survived the Sunday service, now I'll go home and collapse. It was too much 'happy' emotion while I'm dealing with so much."

Another mom, Carol Kent, famous Christian author and speaker, also had to survive a Mother's Day service. It was in the year 2000. The previous year, her life had changed forever when her twenty-five-year-old son, a graduate of the U.S. Naval Academy and a lieutenant in the navy with an impeccable military record, shot and killed his wife's ex-husband.

That Sunday afternoon Carol waited to hear the voice of her only child. She was waiting for a call from prison. It never came. Tears trickled and then flowed as she walked over to her sofa, picked up a light beige afghan her mother had made, hunkered down on the sofa, and covered herself from her neck to her toes. As she sobbed, she cried to God, "I am so broken, hurting, and unable to find peace on this day when other mothers are hugging their children. . . ." Her pain continued to pour as she wept, "I just want to quit living. I am weary of this pain that never goes away. Please rescue me . . . *if you do not remove me from this place of hurt, will you please climb inside this afghan with me and hold me?*" (Emphasis mine.)

She leaned over, reached for her Bible, and turned to a familiar passage. As she read, the words of her Father reassured her of his constant care as he "held on to her."

Read Carol's heart-wrenching story *When I Lay My Isaac Down, Unshakable Faith in Unthinkable Circumstances*. It's written in a minor key, but it gives major hope. It encourages faith and gives hope to many different unthinkable circumstances.

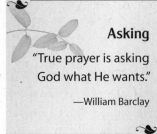

Asking

"True prayer is asking God what He wants."

—William Barclay

Thanks Giving on Thanksgiving

"Giving thanks on Thanksgiving? A few years ago, that was easy. We repeated the usual God-is-great-God-is-good-and-we-thank-him-for-our-food-amen prayer. The table groaned with plates full of food, extended family members crowded around the table, and good health was a given. Giving thanks was easy," a mom said.

"This year we spent Thanksgiving in the hospital room and ate off the tray next to my child's bed. Our smaller immediate family sat on our child's bed, on a recliner, and at the foot of the bed-sofa. Some volunteers brought in a Thanksgiving meal for everyone on the floor, so the smells and tastes made it feel like Thanksgiving.

"We thought back to that first Thanksgiving and the pilgrims who'd spent two months crossing an ocean rocked by storms and landed in the dead of winter. The rest were weak and wouldn't have made it if the Wampanoag Indians hadn't taught them how to plant, hunt, and survive. They shared a bountiful meal and were thankful for food, friends, and health—the basics. "

And there we sat in our CK's room and deeply appreciated our food, friends, and staff and volunteers, and the health that we had at that present time—the basics—nothing taken for granted. Our prayer came deep from within, an appreciation of all we had, and to our Lord who gives us our 'daily bread.' We now thank him for the easy times—and his being with us in the difficult ones."

Merry Christmas!

As a "cancer family," you may have a clearer vision of Christmas than the rest of the world. Carols sung about the midnight sky when angels burst forth on the scene and the way the shepherds froze in fear. The angels had to reassure them, "Fear not. . . ."

Today you may be frozen in fear and need reassuring. But just as the angels proclaimed over two thousand years ago, "Fear not, for behold we bring you good tidings of great joy." That joy came from heaven to earth in the form of a baby.

Read the story for yourself in Luke 2, and then for a modern-day twist, read the humorous paperback *The Best Christmas Pageant Ever* by Barbara Robinson. The Herdmans—a family with six children, considered the town terrors—take over the annual church Christmas pageant with surprising results, for both the town and the Herdmans.

Children, whether fictional like the Herdmans, or real, view Christmas in unique ways that adults sometimes miss. Ethan, a three-year-old CK, brought new meaning to his family on Christmas. His family tells the story:

"We brought down some of the Christmas decorations last week and Ethan found the stockings that hang over the fireplace. He was really excited and interested in the stockings, so we all hung them as we have for years. However, Ethan went back to the box containing the stockings and found an extra one that had never been used.

"He picked it up and said, 'We need to hang this one for Jesus. I think that he would like having a stocking.' We didn't hesitate to hang the extra stocking on the fireplace.

"Once the stocking was up, he said, 'I want to make a heart out of paper and put it in the stocking for Jesus on Christmas.' We promptly helped him cut out a paper heart that he immediately wrote his name on, and then he carefully slipped it into the stocking.

"At that point, we realized that once again the three-year-old in the family taught the adults about life and Christmas.

"All God really wants from us at this time of year is our heart. In fact, that is what he wants from us all year long. We definitely have a new tradition and a reminder of the true meaning of Christmas."

What traditions do you have in your family? It can be hard to keep up with Christmas traditions when you're living in the new normal. Consider which ones are most important to your CK and your other children and maintain those traditions. Think about whether the new normal demands some new traditions.

The Flocks Have Landed

You're heading home. One mom said, "When we got the word that we'd been discharged, we were so excited. We were headed home! Home to my own bed, and my child in her bed. Home with my family, my routines, my washing machine, my neighbors, my refrigerator, my bathroom. . . . I was truly excited. Then I remembered what another mom had told me—that the transition to home isn't necessarily easy.

That mom said, I was so glad to be going home, I never thought about the downside. I had to put back all the stuff that made the hospital room home and then clean up what hadn't been done while I'd been gone. And you know what else? I missed the professionals down the hall. Even in a house full of people, I felt all alone."

A single mom said, "I second-guessed my child's coughs, fever, everything. I was used to the nurses checking in every few hours. I know I can call the nurse at night but I feel like I'm doing that too much already, even though they say I'm not. I thought I'd feel relieved to be home, and I am, but at first I felt overwhelmed. It just seemed to be up to me 24/7 to know what to do. Who am I going to ask for help in the middle of the night, my other preschool children? But I really am glad to be home."

When you get home, you not only deal with fear and second guessing, you may miss your new hospital family. "I miss the families we've met on the floor, and wonder how they are doing. I just need to take the time and call them. And the hospital staff have become some of my best friends. I miss being a part of their lives. Sometimes I just call at three in the afternoon and ask what they're doing. I know that sounds silly, but I still feel connected to them."

It may seem strange that there is an adjustment involved in coming home, but many families find that to be the case. You're not alone. You adjust to the downside and deal with settling in, and then you can appreciate the positives. You're home! You've completed another step on the journey. Your new normal continues to unfold, and your family is back under one roof continuing that journey. Your family is glad you're home, especially those siblings.

*Each day of our lives we make deposits
in the memory banks of our children.*

—Charles Swindoll

Siblings: The Well Ones

There are over 12,000 children diagnosed with cancer each year in the United States, and 270,000-plus childhood cancer survivors. There are at least that many children thrust into the cancer arena with them—their siblings—the well ones. Both are victims of cancer, which affects the rest of their lives. They're on the same road, "But miles apart," a sibling said. We want this chapter to help bring the family closer together.

Siblings are not small adults; they are children, with childlike perspectives and needs. It's easy to shove a teen sibling into the adult role in your family—but they aren't adults—they just look that way. Siblings, whatever age, communicate in various ways with the CK.

McDonalds

Overheard from a preschool sibling: "My mommy lives with Ronald McDonald in his house now."

When Joseph, a teen CK, was asked how his teen sister had treated him during his battle with cancer, he answered, "She acted normal, not like I was sick or anything. We get along pretty well anyway." Then he paused and added, "I guess if your sibling was mean before you got cancer, then they'd need to act better—not normal."

And some do act normal. Seven-year-old James and his six-year-old brother Chad were rolling around on the floor. It looked like a regular sibling fight until Chad yelled at his mom, "What are his counts?" The answer would determine (in his mind) whether he could hit his brother or not. That question brought their mom running into the room—knowing what the normal result would be.

Siblings are individuals with unique personalities, interests, and their own place in your family's birth order. Siblings need help to cope and carve out their own identity. It's important to be more than just "John's brother."

Parents, do whatever it takes to keep communication open with these siblings. Remember that each of you see things from your side of the fence.

Let's listen to some viewpoints from the siblings' side of the fence:

- "My parents' world is now Tiffany. All the rest of us have to stand in line—way down the line. . . ."
- "He's the one who's sick. Why do I feel like I'm the burden? Dad's a zombie and Mom's weepy."

- "I feel invisible. People just look past or through me, or always just ask about my sister. I'm still here, aren't I?"

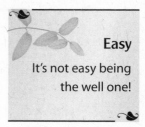

Easy

It's not easy being the well one!

Now let's hear from the parents:

- "Cancer siblings are a wealth of misinformation. I'd never have guessed what they were thinking, not in a million years."
- "I can't meet all their needs. Most of the time, I don't even know what those needs really are. I just live on guilt."
- "As long as the sibling doesn't demand attention, we think everything's okay. I wish that were true."

Opening the Gate

What are the keys to unlock the gate in that fence? Communication is *the* key. Do all you can to keep it as open as possible.

Keep in mind that communication is only eight percent verbal. The other ninety-two percent of communication is body language, eye contact, and tone of voice. Your concern for your child is caught not taught.

Now, be honest from the start. That way, they can trust your word later. Use the word *cancer*; it's floating all over the place. You may feel like that will frighten your children, but you can find the right words. Let children know that cancer is a serious disease, but it does not necessarily mean the person will die from it. One mom said, "Our dear friend [an adult] had cancer, but our four-year-old son told everyone, 'Mine is okay. I have kids' cancer and I'll be fine when I'm seven.'" If you have trouble figuring out the right things to tell the siblings, ask the professionals. They've been through this with other families and they know how to help.

A sibling said, "My parents say, 'He's fine,' and my CK brother says so too. If he's so fine, why is he throwing up all the time?"

Siblings needs more than a quick "He's fine," so plan ahead what you will tell them. They need information to help them understand what's going on.

That's why communication isn't a one-time event. It's much more than just delivering the diagnosis. Keep sibs in the loop on their level. At times you might need to say something like this: "You probably noticed that John is really tired and grumpy lately. The medicines make him that way for right now. What do you think we could do to help him?"

Think about how important good information is to you. The adults in the family are usually processing information. Children need information to process also. Processing and talking through feelings is healthy for everyone. You may not realize how far down the road you have come, and without some information, children may be just beginning to deal with this new difficult journey.

Also, listen for misunderstandings. One dad overheard his son say, "My sister has 'bone arrows' in her back." (He meant "bone marrow.") Explain procedures on the sib's level.

Young children especially need to be reassured they did not cause the cancer in any way—even if they've had "bad" thoughts and actions in the past against the CK. Also, let them know that cancer is not contagious. Some adults may even think that. If needed, contact alternative support people (child life specialists, teachers, chaplains, or church staff) for children to talk to. It may be easier to share feelings, especially negative ones concerning the family, with a neutral third party. They may need to vent at times.

Encourage your children to ask questions. Older children may even want to ask questions of the medical staff. Younger children may draw pictures, and then you can ask them to tell you about the picture. This is a great conversation starter.

A teen sibling said, "A lot of attention is given to my brother, but life is precious and it's his time—so that's okay."

Widening the Circle

Try to make sure the sibs don't miss school and their activities. Difficulties can arise with their friends because they can't relate to the cancer experience. To make matters worse, you are less available to transport the siblings to visit friends or to other activities. Do what you can to facilitate their usual routines and activities. The usual people, places, and routines give "normalcy" to the day and provide a source of support for your children.

Communication is needed with teachers, coaches, and anyone who works with your CK's siblings. Forewarned is forearmed. Talk with them to make sure they are aware of your family's situation. Or if you need to have an assigned friend do this, let the teachers and others know that in writing, in an email, or by phone.

Continue to keep teachers and coaches in the loop with e-mails or notes. Let them know what they can do to help. It's better to take a proactive approach instead of just reacting to the problems. Siblings' reaction to the cancer stress may erupt in negative forms: anger, not doing work, pouting, withdrawing, and crying. All reactions depend on their personalities and how things have been handled in their lives. However, it's also possible for the siblings to demonstrate extremely positive behavior: stuffing negative feelings, overly conscientious, taking on extra responsibilities, and not wanting to add more burdens to the family.

Let teachers and coaches know that you need to know from them what is happening with the siblings. They may say, "But you just have so much on you already." Express your appreciation, but explain that you can't help fix something if you don't know it's broken—that includes behavior and homework. Because of extreme stress, a sibling may need help—and she probably wants one-on-one time with her parents. During certain stages with your CK, you may not be able to give that time to the siblings. Include other adults in your children's lives and be appreciative of their involvement in your children's world. Just a brief note of thanks will make their day. These people play a crucial role and they're a positive piece of the puzzle. Let them know that.

Daily Routines

Routines create a sense of security for children as their world has flipped upside down. Talk about regular routines; ask what they really miss that isn't happening now. You may be surprised how insignificant that routine may seem to you as an adult, but how important it is to the children. Review the "Love Languages" at the end of Resource One for clues as to why certain things are important to them.

The new normal includes a new routine, but it may be constantly changing. Explain any necessary changes that have to come into these new ravaged routines. Also, let the children know there may be changes that you can't let them know about beforehand, but you'll have a special time to talk with them afterwards. Transitions are especially difficult for introverted Blues (see Resource One), "But we always read a story before bedtime," he may say. His very outgoing Yellow sibling probably won't care about transitions and changes as long as there are still people around to talk to.

Again, this is the new normal. Allow children to find ways to help and be included in the family's new routines. You can encourage the children by saying: "Things are not like they were before cancer—when things were normal. But we now have a new normal and all of us will plan how we live it. We're in this together."

Try to be as positive as possible. They'll pick up on your attitude.

Acknowledge when their perceptions and thoughts are correct about what is happening in your CK's life and your family's life. They'll be able to trust their thoughts and ideas later in life as you reinforce them during this trying time. Many children feel that adults never listen to their ideas and opinions.

Encourage your children to participate in the care of their CK sibling, both at home and in the hospital.

Let's Pray for Those Involved

Lord,

Thank you for all those involved in my child(ren)'s life. Give them wisdom, love, and strength for all the duties they have and all the lives they touch.

Amen.

Decisions

Many families' routines include a bright, orange-haired clown.

Pulling into the McDonald's parking lot, siblings may point to the CK and say, "What are his counts?" Meaning, "Can we go inside to play—not just hit the drive-thru?" Answers to "What are his counts?" determine decisions in the new normal.

However, be careful not to put additional, unnecessary responsibility on the older ones or those who will say yes to whatever is asked.

If possible, allow children to attend some clinic or hospital visits so that they can get to know the staff and receive some encouragement from them. Siblings can also spend time with their CK sister or brother in the hospital playing games, watching TV, and just spending quality time together. Some may want to do that, and some may not. "He wants to act like nothing is going on. That's his way of coping," one mom said about her CK's brother.

When a CK came home from the hospital with her cards, toys, and games as well as mom's full attention, a sibling said, "I thought when my sister came home we'd go back to our normal routines, like before the cancer. Now it's even more real because she's in the next room, and back in school, and the expression 'new normal' sure is true! Our routines completely revolve around her, and I wish I wasn't so resentful."

Emotional Landmines

Allow yourself to express your emotions in front of your children—to a certain point, depending on their ages and personalities. This delivers an important message: Mom gets frustrated and cries at times, so I can too. Catharsis, which is a feeling of release of an intense emotional experience, is important on this journey. Encourage your children to express their emotions openly and honestly with you. You both need a good catharsis.

However, the majority of the time you should let your children see a smile on your face—even if it is a forced smile. Still better, watch a funny movie together and laugh. Endorphins kick in and all of you need that.

Anger

There's a lot of potential for anger in the new normal. It may sound like this when it comes from your CK's siblings:

- "Do I have to wash my hands all the time and wear those masks?"
- "How long is this trip going to be?"
- "Why can't I just sleep in my own bed?"
- "Grandma doesn't know the cereal I like or the video games I play, and she can't help me with my math. She just sighs a lot."
- "I can't have my friends over cause his counts are too low again."
- "My mom used to be nice. Now, not so much."

What does anger sound like in *your* children? Keep your ears open for it. Here are some tips to help with your children's anger.

- Let children know it is okay to still have fun and do normal activities even though your family is coping with cancer. Remember, laughter is healthy. It's hard to remember that at times, isn't it?

- Encourage your children to write in a journal or diary or draw pictures. This can provide a safe place for them to express their anger. (It can help them work through other negative emotions also.)
- Encourage physical activity. Have the children run laps around your yard, shoot baskets, or climb on a playground. They need to work through their feelings and concerns—not bottle them up. You do too, by the way.
- Maintain consistent discipline with all of your children (no matter what the negative reactions are). Boundaries give the stability they all need.

Jealousy

Siblings may think, "He gets everything, even mom." Then the guilt kicks in and the next thought may be, "How could I think that?" One sibling said, "How do you live up to 'the legend' who has so much courage? I can never be what he is."

Jealousy may look like this: your CK has been throwing up for hours and then your well one throws up a little. Your CK is fatigued, and then your well one is tired all the time and wants to cuddle. It's past midnight and your CK is wired on steroids, you pop in a DVD to pass the time, and guess who shows up at the bedroom door? "I just can't sleep," the well one mumbles. "But those actions are psychosomatic. They're not real," one mom said. The truth is that they are very real to the sufferer. If

Blankets

If your CK has received a warm fleecy blanket or quilt, each sibling may need a special one too.

A blanket can be comforting at any age.

you encounter a situation like that, do whatever it takes to spend time with the sib. Say, "I'm so sorry you don't feel well. Let's wrap you in this quilt and snuggle. What would taste good to you?" The cure for jealousy is time and attention. Even small doses help.

> **Sibling Thoughts**
>
> "I feel invisible. People just look past or through me, or always just ask about my sister. I'm still here, aren't I?"

Frustration

We asked many siblings what advice or tips they would give to other siblings. The answer? "One word: PATIENCE! Know that you aren't in the spotlight, at all. That your parents are doing the best they can, and are probably worried about finances, jobs, and having to deal with a child with cancer. Just have patience."

"People grab your arm at church, school, everywhere and say, 'How is he doing?' I don't really like to have my arm grabbed all the time, but I've learned to just smile, give them a short, planned answer and say, 'Thank you for asking.'"

Another sib said, "Everyone says, 'How are you doing?' I feel like saying, 'Lousy! How are you doing?' Actually, that isn't totally true. The people who've gone through this say other things. I can't remember what they are; just that it doesn't make me mad."

Talking to a child life specialist or counselor may also alleviate a child's concerns or frustrations. Again, it may help him cope and carve out his own identity—not just "John's brother."

Embarrassment

A sibling confessed, "My sister has a bald head, a bloated round face, and circles under her eyes. People stare and I just get embarrassed. Then I feel guilty for feeling embarrassed. She's my sister, and going through—well, I can't say the word."

If you sense a sibling may be dealing with this, offer your help. Encourage the sibling to talk through these feelings. Do it without condemnation, which means watch your body language. No sighing, shaking your head, or clicking your tongue.

Validate the sibling's feelings. They're real.

Loneliness

An older sibling may spend many hours home alone. She may be microwaving meals by herself. If grandma and friends come in it helps, but not always. The older sibling may be torn between "I don't need a babysitter" and feeling like nothing can replace the family that is usually there. Take time to talk to these "almost adults" about their feelings.

Keep the siblings (whatever age) with you as a family as much as possible. Sharing Jell-O on a hospital tray beats anything anywhere at times. Reassure your children that they will be cared for no matter what happens. You may feel that they surely know that—but they don't. Cancer has thrown everything into upheaval, and mainly they just want you—no matter what their age.

Fear

The underlying emotion in most siblings is fear. Fear of CK's condition and death; fear that parents may get sick and die; fear that they will be left alone. Assure them (repeatedly) that someone will always be there to take care of them.

Filling the Tanks

Show your children that you love them by filling those tanks again—and again and again. What are their love languages? (Review the end of Resource One.) Here are some ways to show your love and fill those emotional tanks:

- **Touch.** This includes hugs for teens too.
- **Time.** Stop, look (eye to eye), and listen. Don't just mumble, "Uh huh." Ask where the sib would like to spend time with you.
- **Talk.** Encouraging words give courage to keep on keeping on. They may get daily doses of discouraging words in life.
- **Gifts.** Not particularly expensive. Just something to say, "I'm thinking about you." Choose something meaningful just for them.
- **Deeds.** What do the children do? Thank them for those acts, and find things to do for them.

When we asked sibs, "What was a big help to your family?" many said the same thing. "People brought food!" Deeds done in love. We all need to receive those.

Two more helpful books by Gary Chapman are *Five Love Languages of Children* and *Five Love Languages of Teenagers*. They make good reading in the middle of the night.

❧ ❧ ❧

Dear Reader, as you hold this book in your hands, rest assured you have been prayed for by the authors and fellow travelers. You and your family are important to us.

We pray that these words encourage you as you affect the lives of your children—cancer kids and well ones. We pray that God will sweep away the fog, give you clarity to view each child, and strength to meet those needs—one step at a time.

Again, you are precious to us and more so to him. He is the one who gives us others who come alongside.

Some people come into our lives and quickly go. Some stay for awhile and leave footprints on our hearts. And we are never, ever the same.

—Anonymous

Friends:
The Family You Choose

One mom said, "You know she's a real friend when she calls to ask how your child's counts are before scheduling her child's birthday party." Another one added, "Friends know when your child's next treatment is, and what that entails—even flushing a port."

Like an elastic bandage wrapped snuggly around a sprained ankle, giving support during the healing process, friends wrap around you and provide support during your healing process. Friends don't squeeze too tight and smother you, but they do give you strength as you continue to function. Allow them that privilege. Don't let them miss the blessing.

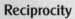

Reciprocity

Friends help increase endorphins in your brain. And friendships help increase the endorphins in your friend's brain also. It goes both ways.

Friends are "family," not by blood or marriage, but by love. Sometimes they're closer than relatives in location and in relationships. They help you carry the burden and get the job done.

Friends offer support just as family does. They bring so many positives into a difficult situation. Many parents noted that friends bring food, pick up the kids, transport the siblings to and from extracurricular activities, and take them out for fun. Friends also provide spiritual support and prayer.

One mom said, "No matter how bad things have gotten, just being with these church 'sisters' helps me remember that this world isn't the end." Another said, "I have to set limits on how long I unload on some friends. I can completely drain them without realizing it."

A Gift That Keeps On Giving
—Lynda and Donna

In the clinic waiting room, Donna and I leaned back on the sofa. Across the room, sat her fourteen-year-old son, Trevor, diagnosed with cancer two years ago. He was now in remission and was here assisting the volunteer art therapist. I leaned toward Donna and asked, "With all you've been through, do you have a favorite scripture that's helped?"

Donna thought a moment, and then glanced down at her wrist, and slowly turned her silver bracelet. "One is the verse on this bracelet. Our close friend who had had a brain tumor gave it to me. The tumor appeared twenty years ago, and she'd been in remission these last seven years. Then it came back." Donna paused. "She passed away eighteen months ago."

"I'm so sorry."

She took off the bracelet, placed it in my hand, and continued, "I always felt like God left her here all those years to help Trevor when we went through this terrible time."

Reminders of Love

Do you have a visual reminder of a friend's love and faith? Drop a thank you note, another visual reminder of love that keeps on giving.

I fingered the engraved hearts and flowers, and silently read the verse, "In all your ways acknowledge Him, And He shall direct your paths" (Prov. 3:6).

"This is so beautiful, Donna."

"That's Trevor's favorite verse too. He really misses her. I can't begin to tell you all the ways she helped us."

I handed her back the bracelet, and she slipped it on her wrist. With a faint smile, she said, "Every time I look at it I think of her and her faith. It just keeps on giving."

Has a friend given you a visual reminder of his or her love and faith? Drop them a thank you note, another visual reminder of love that keeps on giving.

Pastor Kelvin's Job Description
—Lynda and Hedy

I tapped softly on the hospital room door. After a whispered, "Come in," I slowly opened it. What a tender sight. In the recliner sat eight-year-old Danielle on the lap of a young man, her bald head resting on his shoulder. He continued reading a book to her as she slipped in and out of drug-induced sleep. The softness of this picture provided a sharp contrast to the steel IV pole standing by the chair.

Her mom, Hedy, waved me in. "This is Pastor Kelvin, our children's minister from church. Danielle just loves him and his wife, Carol."

Pastor Kelvin smiled.

"Wish I could take a picture of this," I said, as I shook his hand around Danielle's sleeping body.

Later I heard stories of Danielle in Carol's children's choir at church.

"The first week Danielle was in choir, Carol heard someone singing with all their might. It was coming from Danielle. Danielle who'd been in the hospital fighting cancer!" Kelvin said. He chuckled, looked down at her peaceful face, and said, "Whatever she does, she does a hundred percent."

His job, visiting children in the hospital, usually dealt with tonsils and broken legs—not with critical illnesses. A new part of his ministry had begun, an extremely difficult one, but a blessed part that would change him forever.

He said later, "I look at healthcare professionals in a different light now. This is their passion, to do this kind of work. I look them in the eye and say I appreciate them, and for them to pass the thanks on to the others."

Carol and Kelvin continue living out the following verse: "Therefore comfort each other and edify one another, just as you also are doing" (1 Thess. 5:11).

Root Wrapping

Majestic redwoods grow in groups of five and their shallow roots intertwine. This enables trees to survive severe storms. Like redwoods, cancer families root wrap, enabling them to survive severe storms. Root wrapping starts in waiting rooms. It continues in hospital halls, support groups, chat rooms, e-mails, and phone calls.

"I hate to say to the new parents on the floor, 'Welcome to the club that none of us wanted to join,'" said a mom. "It's a bizarre world with a secret language. And you know you've joined the club when these words flow out of your mouth and they sound logical: . . . the EMLA cream takes about an hour to work . . . they'll flush the port . . . then may start the Methotrexae. . . ."

Here's what some parents say about the club that no one wanted to join:

- "There's no president, it's all equal opportunity, no matter what you have or don't have. Some families are wealthy; some have absolutely nothing of this world's goods. But all families feel the same help-lessness when they hear the diagnosis. One family included a child (Robin Bush) whose father would become president of the United States, and later her older brother also—no one is immune."
- "There's no secretary, but you need to keep your own daily journal including meds, reactions to the meds, and helpful hints for hospital staff caring for your child. You are your child's best advocate."
- "There's no treasurer, all the money is out-go, not income—except from generous friends and organizations. Ask the social workers and other professionals at the hospital to help you locate organizations and help if needed."

- "No one ever looks forward to welcoming new members; we hope our club will become extinct."

Once you're admitted, you have a lifetime membership in the club. The upside of that is you have others who really understand and encourage you (which helps you endure being in the club).

Some of you have just joined this club, others have been members a short while, and others for as long as you can remember.

Whatever length of time, please take advantage of others in the club. They're there for you—night and day. "It's amazing how giving brings such huge returns. We don't do it for that, but it just works that way. Welcome to the club."

Root Wrapping Continues
—Lynda and Hedy

As I passed the oncology family waiting room, there was Hedy. She's never out of Danielle's room. I popped my head in the door, "What are you doing in here?"

"Danielle went for tests, but I couldn't go with her this time." She turned to a lady standing nearby and added, "I want you to meet my new friend, Virginia. Her teenage son Jeremy has just been diagnosed."

I clasped her hand, "I'm so glad to meet you, Virginia."

"Me too," she said and set her coffee on the counter. We hugged. (That's done a lot on this floor.)

"Do you have time to talk for a little while?" Hedy asked.

I glanced at my list of patients in need of bedside tutoring. I'd made it

> **Forever**
>
> Who are the adults touching your child's life? They'll be changed forever.

through the list. "I can't believe it, but I'm finished."

The three of us sat on the sofas and leaned in to talk over the TV's chatter.

"Virginia, tell me about your son," I said.

"He was diagnosed not that long ago, after many misdiagnoses." She continued with the details of his disease, and then she said, "With teen boys you worry about drugs or car accidents. It never entered our minds to worry about cancer. When we found out, we were overwhelmed and I just couldn't breathe. It's been several weeks now, and it's finally soaking in."

> **God's Promise**
>
> Let each of you look out not only for his own interests, but also for the interests of others.
>
> —Philippians 2:4

"How's he doing?"

She leaned back, crossed her arms, and said, "He's doing as well as can be expected. He's a real fighter, but you know, this sounds crazy, even though we're totally drained, we've prayed and come to a peace about this—whatever happens."

As the hour went on, Hedy and Virginia talked about their children. So much about their children was different—diagnosis, age, and gender—but the horrendous journey was the same.

Hedy then turned to me and asked, "So how is your son doing?"

I didn't want to talk about my "healthy" son. After my quick, "He's fine," Hedy told Virginia his story—about his family of six living in a motel room for months. I was amazed to then find myself talking about his teen years—drugs and all—and about God completely turning his life around.

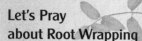

Let's Pray about Root Wrapping

Thank you, Lord, for those you've led into my life and allowed us to root wrap. Show me others whose roots need wrapping.

"Oh my goodness," Virginia exclaimed. "I could never have dealt with drugs with Jeremy. That must have been awful."

I sat there amazed. "Drugs worse than cancer?" I asked.

"For me, yes. I don't think I could have handled that."

Hedy added, "God really does give us grace for whatever we're going through, and we've had some different journeys, haven't we?"

We nodded, joined hands, and gave a quick squeeze.

Hedy glanced at her watch. "I've got to get back to the room. She'll be coming back from the tests, but I want you both to know how this has blessed me."

"God just keeps putting people in my life here. . . ." Virginia's voice trailed off.

We hugged again, and I said, "I still can't believe you weren't in Danielle's room."

"I know. This was one of the few times I wasn't able to go with her for tests. So, I came here for coffee—and met Virginia," she said, taking her arm. "And here you came by. What coincidences."

Like Hedy and Virginia, you may find that your roots often wrap with new people. On another day, shortly after I met Virginia, I was passing by the family waiting room again. Virginia and I spotted each other, and I was privileged to meet another one of their kindred spirits—Tracey.

"Virginia's been such a help with the financial information she's learned. Guess everyone on this floor could use that advice," said Tracey.

Days later, I sat across the table at a fast food restaurant with Tracey and her husband, Bob, as they poured out their story. Their difficult journey began before their son Jay's cancer diagnosis—several years before. Overwhelming financial burdens flooded their lives after a job layoff.

"We didn't even have money for gas to get to church, so we'd simply pray for it, dig behind cushions on the sofa, scrounge in the floorboard of the car, and come up with quarters. We'd yell, 'Thank you, Lord,' then head out to get the gas—whatever those quarters would buy," Bob said. "I really think the hard years we went through and his faithfulness to supply our needs prepared us for this most difficult part of our lives."

"Another thing," said Tracey. "A year before Jay's cancer, we were burdened to pray for seven friends with cancer. Little did we know . . ." She pushed her food on her plate with her fork. "And you never know what someone else is going through. You have to keep your eyes open, even when you're going through your own problems."

Bob added, "Some people you've got to meet are the Lees from our church. Their teenage son, Joseph, had cancer before Jay, and he's been such an inspiration to our family. They brought us parking passes,

God's Promise

Blessed be the . . . God of all comfort, who comforts us in all our tribulation, that we may be able to comfort those who are in any trouble, with the comfort with which we ourselves are comforted by God.

—2 Corinthians 1:3-4

Jolly Ranchers ® for Jay's sore throat, caps for his head, and lots of advice."

The root wrapping goes on and on and on. . . .

Take a few moments to think about the coincidences God has brought into your life on this journey. Who are the new friends you're root wrapping with? What have they done for you? What have you had the opportunity to do for them? Thank him for his coincidences—and for all the others God will bring into your life, and your CK's life, in the future. Now meet more new friends in the new place.

*At the timberline where the storms strike
with most fury, the sturdiest trees are found.*

—Hudson Taylor

Hospital Hospital–ity

I visited my friend in the hospital and glanced down at her room number written on a slip of paper. At the bottom was stamped: Quiet please. *Healing in progress.*

Yes, healing is in progress—in more ways than we know. Healing is dispensed, not only in the pharmacy, but also through the staff as they meet needs: physical, emotional, and spiritual. How do you react to the staff and *their* needs?

"My child is so sick, how can I think of anyone else?" Overwhelmed parents may have little patience in dealing with the humanness in hospital staffs. However, hospital staffs are human. They have their own families, health issues, and stress factors—not the least is working in a children's hospital. As you interact with these new people in the new place, review Resource

Humor Helps

Females are females are females:
In your CK's hospital room, mix one nurse with PMS cramps, add one peri-menopausal mom hissing, "What mood swings!?" Then top it off with one menopausal grandmother furiously fanning and wiping sweat from her upper lip and hairline.

One on personalities, which will help you understand them better as individuals. Remember that you're all on the same team, working toward the same goal—to help your child.

You know how frustrated you feel when you ask the doctors your why questions and they reply, "We don't really know why." On the other side of that fence, they too want to know the answer to the whys, and they devote their lives to finding those answers. They deal with the whys every day. Your pain is their pain, too.

Around tables at staff meetings and grabbing one-on-one sessions in the hall, these professionals wrestle with difficult questions and plans of action in a field where there are few guideposts and fewer guarantees. Some smile, give hugs, and shed tears with you; others appear reserved and only give objective answers. Some days your smile may not be returned, but keep giving it away. You never know what is happening in someone else's life. Healthcare professionals are human first and professionals second.

In 2005, after hurricane Katrina devastated the gulf coast, the New Orleans Children's Hospital posted this page on their website. It spoke volumes.

"Everyone continues to put all of the personal loss behind them and tend to the patients, our first priority. It is only in the silence of a broken heart, when alone for a few minutes, or with a trusted co-worker, that the tears flow briefly, and then it is back to business. I do believe that most of the patients do not know the extent of the loss of the healthcare workers that are caring for them. And, they shouldn't know it. It should not be their burden."

A Hospital Tour

Welcome to a children's hospital: kid-sized and child friendly! As you enter the doors, you're bombarded by vibrant colors splashed across the walls, ceiling, floors, doors, and chairs. Red wagons and wheelchairs, along with IV poles and pumps, are maneuvered through the mazelike halls by parents, siblings, volunteers, and staff. Each hospital is unique, but the same in the most important way. They all state, "We're here for each child."

As you meet the staff along the way, give them a huge gift—a smile! This is especially needed if they're not wearing one. They may not have seen one in a long time, as each of their days is stitched with concern for all the children in their care.

Another huge gift to give staff is to pray for them each day. Pray for wisdom as they make decisions affecting the children in their care, and pray for them and their families. God knows their individual needs.

Who are the people on the staff? Keep your eyes open.

Parking Garage

The mom drove into the hospital's parking garage, came to a stop, and pushed the familiar ticket button. She pulled the ticket from the machine, the yellow-striped security arm rose, and she began the ascent. Level 1A, slowly circling; 1B, no spots; 2A, circle; 2B, not anything yet; 3A, 3B, someone pulling out?; 4A, 4B, 5A, 5B, 6A, last chance before the off-limits helicopter pad; 6A, an open spot!

Mom unharnessed her sleeping child from the car seat, lifted his slumping weight, and shifted him on to her shoulder. Then she grabbed the diaper bag (which served as a carryall) and threw it over her other shoulder, balancing herself out.

She trudged to the elevator, pushed the button, and waited—and waited. Thus began another day dealing with a gamut of people and procedures. Today she was headed toward the clinic—where waiting had become an art form.

Information Desk

Stepping out of the elevator, many families need assistance with directions. Help usually is nearby—information and a smile—delivered from the information desk.

One person who worked the information desk said, "People wander off the elevators with that lost look. They think they should know answers to simple questions, but many don't. Everything is scary and new, but it's old to us. Their minds are crowded with concerns for their child, and they just need a friendly face to let them know we're here to help. I'm blessed to come alongside these people each day.

"One day a mommy just stood there and cried, and as we talked, no phones rang! That had to be God working. My husband said I have a Kleenex ministry."

Tips 'n' Tricks

Be especially careful in your home away from home—your vehicle.

Hours spent on the road driving to and from the hospital, clinic, and home can be hazardous when you're weary.

Pay special attention to rain-slicked or snow-covered streets.

And watch speed limits. (A 35 MPH speed limit doesn't change to 65 MPH in the middle of the night.)

These people answer questions and attempt to listen—between umpteen phone calls.

One staffer said, "If we can alleviate any of their trauma, then we've done our job. And we want them to know that as long as there's life, there's hope." Those who work the information desk stand at the ready to help with anything.

One day I stopped by to give a young girl her bedside tutoring in the intensive care unit (ICU). The mom said, "We've been in this room for six weeks, and today I got caught in the bathroom. The door wouldn't open and I kept banging on it and yelling to my daughter to call the nurse. She didn't do it because she thought I was joking. Would you joke about that? I don't know who to call to come fix that door."

"Let me make a quick call to the information desk. She'll know who to contact," I said. Minutes later, maintenance came and fixed the doorknob.

A year later, I sat at my dining room table with my friend Hedy and her friend Faye—both had recently lost their daughters to cancer. We talked about their lives, and suddenly Faye mentioned being in ICU for weeks at a time. It clicked.

"You weren't stuck in the bathroom once, were you?" I asked.

"How did you know?"

"I was that volunteer from the schoolroom."

"You called the information lady and she got the door fixed!"

Small world. Small hospital world.

Chaplains

According to the dictionary, a chaplain is a member of the clergy employed to give religious guidance, but they do much more than that. One of their more important roles it to offer a kind, listening ear. "We had no choice in this horrendous journey, but they [chaplains] choose to enter our pain," a CK's mom said. "And we are privileged to do so," the chaplain responded. Chaplains are usually the first line of spiritual help in the hospital, ministering to patients, parents, and staff.

The following story is told by Chaplain Ward.

At our yearly remembrance service for families of children who had died in the past year, the room continued to fill with staff and families. One by one, the oncology staff vacated their chairs for the grieving families. Finally, the room was packed, every seat taken, and staff lined the walls.

I then said, "Families, look around the room at the staff standing against the walls. I served as a chaplain in the Marine Corps, and those Marines had nothing on these people standing around you. These are the warriors and soldiers who fight for your children every day. They stand here surrounding you, and stand with you at the hospital—a wall of caregivers."

One family member began to clap, more joined, then clapping erupted as families rose to their feet. Later, staff members said, "We knew families appreciated us, but to see an entire room give a standing ovation was overwhelming."

Chaplains minister to groups and to individual families as they serve in the trenches everyday.

Doctors

"I don't know how these doctors (and staff) do this job. I can't imagine choosing to deal with childhood cancer day in and day out," a mom said.

"I don't know how these parents deal with this day in and day out," an oncology staff person replied.

Both appreciate the horrendous task each carries. Both put the child's welfare above their own. Both encourage the other's role in this part of the journey, thereby giving courage to persevere.

One CK's mom said, "When you've hit the wall—again—don't see your doctor as the enemy. Appreciate the responsibilities that he has; he determines the whole course of treatment for your child. Decisions are made by the team, but this person's opinion will shape everything. Doctors' schedules are packed, so do your homework keeping up on new information on the Internet. If you come across more helpful information, ask for a consultation with the doctor. Don't grab the doctor in the hall or when they're making rounds if you need to discuss your child's situation more in depth. Value their time and expertise. You're on the same team. I told our doctor, 'You have my most prized possession [my daughter] in the world.' He said he kept remembering my words. He was our advocate from day one."

How do you relate to the doctors taking care of your child?

Some parents say, "She's the doctor, the professional. I'm just the mom." Keep in mind that you're a team. Your child needs an advocate (you) to keep watch on her meds, feelings (you know her better than anyone), and all the day-by-day issues. Healthcare professionals are human. Many times they are overworked and weary. Occasionally mistakes happen—not on purpose. So you

> **God's Promise**
>
> Be strong and of good courage, do not fear nor be afraid of them; for the LORD your God, He *is* the One who goes with you. He will not leave you nor forsake you.
>
> —Deuteronomy 31:6

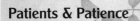

Patients & Patience
Pediatric doctors take care of patients and give patience to parents.

can help them by keeping track in a journal of medications, reactions to those medications, and methods to use. This protects and benefits your child, the staff, and you.

Other parents express a sentiment like this one: "I've never trusted doctors, and you better believe I'm double-checking everything going on. My baby [age seventeen] had a bad reaction to that new medication they gave him. Seems like they'd know better."

All it takes is one outburst or negative comment to undermine your child's confidence in his medical care. You want the best healing situation for him, not the worst. If you have questions, ask them in the hall, not by your child's bedside. And no matter how stressed you are, remember you're addressing a fellow human being who cares about your child—one who is on his care team.

Nurses

Nurses serve on the front line of the battle and few understand the thoughts, feelings, and fears of the patients and families better than they. Each patient's journey is unique in changes and challenges. Every day brings new twists in the road.

One nurse, Mary Ann, tells her story, recounting her days as a pediatric oncology nurse. "I just couldn't understand it. People said, 'We really depend on you as our nurse and appreciate all you do for us.' I loved their children, and this was my job. I just never expected that love to be returned. I always felt that I was the lucky one to have come in contact with these families."

Mary Ann left nursing as her family expanded, and they moved to another state. Then baby number six was born—with a severe heart defect.

"They gave this precious child two years to live," Mary Ann said. "Our world fell apart, and I began to experience life from the other side [as the parent of a critically ill child]. As the nurses came and went out of our room 24/7, I finally understood what the parents years ago were telling me.

"I depended on the nurses and appreciated each small kindness shown to us. It was often the nurses who picked up the pieces when I was left in tears after listening to the doctor and the situation with our child. Being the recipient gave me a whole new appreciation for being a nurse and I'll never forget the nurses who cared for our child."

Mary Ann has experienced both sides, helping and being helped.

Social Worker

One of the computer support staff at the hospital said, "A friend talked me into walking up a small local mountain. Being a veteran climber, she set a pace that I struggled breathless to follow. As the summit came into sight, I stopped to massage my cramping legs and suck in some much needed air. I told her I couldn't finish the hike. She didn't respond the way many people would, by saying, 'Sure you can.' Instead she simply said, 'Give me your hand.'

Needles & Hugs

From a CaringBridge site: "I learned that only a child would greet with a smile, a hug, and a kiss, the person that sticks a needle in their spine once a month. And only an oncology doctor or nurse is deserving of such admiration."

"I gladly accepted her help and her strength, and we finished the climb hand in hand."

Social workers are there to give you a hand, especially when you've reached your limit. When your cramping legs, shortness of breath, and despairing thoughts scream, "Just give up," these professionals extend a hand. They will help you on this journey inside the hospital and outside as you go home. They've been trained to do this. They have climbed this mountain with others, and they are there to give you strength and guidance on this difficult climb.

Grab their hand.

Child Life Specialist

"We're basically 'distracters' who bring toys and sometimes sing to the child during procedures and doctor's appointments," a child life specialist said. "We help the CK and family to learn positive coping skills, and reduce anxiety while going through treatment."

Play, art, and music therapy help children understand their illness and medical procedures. They can express their feelings and simply have fun. "We're also there to help celebrate important events in the child's life, such as birthdays, end of treatment parties, and accomplishing goals set by families and staff."

Outside of their hospital rooms, playrooms and TeenZones are safe, supportive places where patients and siblings can enjoy special activities

> **God's Promise**
>
> *Let* your speech always Be with grace, seasoned with salt, that you may know how you ought to answer each one.
>
> —Colossians 4:6

and entertainment. No medical procedures are allowed in rooms identified as "safe places."

Healthy children experience play as a normal part of life. For ill children, play is even more important; it helps them cope with their overwhelming experiences in the hospital.

The "ists" and "gists"

There are many "ists"—some are therapists, nutritionists, pharmacists—and there are many "gists"—such as oncologists and radiologists. They all play crucial roles in your child's life. Thank the "ists" and the "gists" as they interact with you and your child.

Volunteers

"You've got quite a load in that wagon," a man on the elevator said. The volunteer was delivering a mound of new toys to the children on the third floor.

"You can't give without receiving," she said.

Volunteers give of their time and help with hundreds of tasks to come alongside the hospital staff.

"We'd never be able to do all the things we do without the hundreds of volunteers," said the volunteer coordinator. "They give us extra sets of hands and listening ears, and they give love to the children and their parents. They enjoy bringing smiles to the children's faces—especially to those who seldom smile.

"Some parents and older siblings of CKs and even the CKs themselves want to come back to the hospital to volunteer once their stay is over. They really want to give back," the coordinator explained.

A volunteer who was a retired nurse said, "Things are so different in children's hospitals today. I watched a little boy with a small remote-controlled car weaving serpentine down the hall. The staff gingerly stepped over the car and never complained. I couldn't believe it. Years ago, someone would have grabbed him up and taken him to his room. It's amazing how the staff works around and with the patients."

Educational support

Some children's hospitals have classrooms, schoolteachers, and volunteers. They give normalcy for about three hours, five days a week. The CK feels as if there is a future beyond cancer as he accomplishes tasks, and it pays off later when he returns to school. He's not far behind in his work; maybe he'll even be caught up.

What if the CK just doesn't feel like coming to school? Bedside tutoring can bring school to them—also for BMT patients and others in isolation. This gives parents and other caregivers a break to leave the room while the schoolroom tutor works with the child.

Overwhelmed parents may not think schoolwork is important; there are too many other issues demanding their attention. However, this is something parents and CKs can assert some control over, and controlling anything on this journey is worth the effort.

Furthermore, parents of teens fear that the CK's grade point average will go down if they don't keep up with their studies, and that will affect being accepted into college. CK's fear this too.

Some hospital teachers have this advice to share:

- "Every child needs to go at their own rate, what they can handle. We give an objective input about that."

- "Depending on your county, check and see what rights you are entitled to for getting help with schoolwork. You may be able to get a homebound teacher, if necessary. You will have to be forceful and polite. You are your child's best advocate. Every child is a special needs child here at the hospital."
- "Nurses work with us and wait to give meds causing nausea after the child has been to school. This small act is huge to us and to the child trying to focus and study."
- "In the clinic, 'chairside tutoring' is great. It counts as a day at school, and they don't just veg in front of the TV."
- "When a child comes to the schoolroom, her social skills are honed, and most kids interact as if they were at school.
- "Parents, if you have teachers [resource people], trust and use them. It takes more off your already full plate. That's our job."

Environmental Services —Hedy

Nothing is quite as lonely as your child's hospital room in the evening. You sit and watch your child, watch the IV tubes and bags, and watch the TV with glazed eyes. Your mind is too tired to concentrate. Here's my angel story—disguised with mop and cleaning products.

I'd hit the wall. My prayers went nowhere, I thought. I'd watched my child suffer in pain all day, the meds weren't giving relief, and I just couldn't take it anymore. I dissolved into hot tears. Then I heard this soft voice say, "Excuse me." I raised my head, and

Every Moment

Those who come to clean the rooms are on the journey too.

They observe the extreme pain in lives of children and parents every day as they do their jobs.

One grandfather brightened a custodial staff member's day when he said, "I can't imagine what this room would look like if you didn't do your job!"

wiped my eyes; there was the lady to clean the room. I tried to force a smile, but then she slowly walked over to my chair. She said, "You look like you're havin' a bad time. Can I pray for you?"

That did it—the floodgates opened. She leaned over, wrapped her arms around me, and quietly prayed near my ear. All I could do was weep. Eventually she asked, "Are you going to be okay?"

I replied, "You'll never know what you've done for me tonight. God sent you just when I needed you."

X-ray Technician —Hedy

As I pushed my daughter, Danielle, in her wheelchair and maneuvered her IV pole, I struggled uphill through the gray stucco tunnel that connected the children's hospital with the adult X-ray department. Out of breath and sweating, I finally arrived and wheeled her through the door. I then heard the calmest voice welcome us, and his friendly smile warmed my weary soul. He ushered us into the X-ray room, and I started to hoist Danielle on to the table with my last amount of strength. The technician gently took her from my arms. I pulled Danielle back and I insisted, "Thank you, but I can do this."

"I've got her, Mom," he said, and he gently placed her on the table. He focused his attention on her and started kidding with her.

My tears came to the surface, not just from weariness, but more so from his kindness. After the x-rays were finished, he lifted her from the metal table and placed her back into the wheelchair as she chose a prize from the familiar bowl that sat on the table. He then leaned over to her and whispered, "Danielle, go ahead and take more prizes."

She smiled, fingered several small toys, and placed the chosen ones in her lap. I thanked him again as I guided the wheelchair and IV pole out the door, but I'll never forget how he said, "I've got her Mom." I needed that simple act of gentleness for my daughter, and for her exhausted mom.

Cafeteria

"I need one hand to pull the wagon, and one to steer the IV pole, and one to push my tray. I've run out of hands," the dad said in the cafeteria line. If possible, plan for the cafeteria and places requiring more than two hands to maneuver.

Give those who work there a smile over the steam table or as you hand them money in the check-out line. They watch an endless line of weary families and rushed staff.

Family Resource Center

Whether you're looking for research on your child's disease, a novel for yourself, children's books, DVDs, or a computer to use, these are the people to ask and this is the place to come.

Gift Shop

Necessities, magazines, books, toys, and cards can all be found here. It's

Seasons

"We went into the hospital in the summer, only leaving for short spurts. When we came out in the fall, I wondered why it was so cold. I finally realized I'd missed a season."

probably the only store within walking distance. Take advantage
—it may be your only "outing" for weeks at a time.

Parking Garage—Hedy

Coming back to the hospital after Danielle's death was extremely
painful, everything brought back memories. As I was leaving the
parking garage for the last time, I slowly drove down each level
and stopped on the first floor at the ticket booth. I rolled down
my window and handed the young woman my ticket and money.

She smiled and said, "Well, hi there. I haven't seen you in a
while. How's your daughter doing?"

I wasn't expecting that. Here was someone I saw for two
years as I parked in this garage, but she was someone who hadn't
heard. So I said, "Thank you so much for asking, but she passed
away a few weeks ago."

The shocked, sad look on her face said it all. Then she whispered, "Oh, I'm so sorry."

I knew she meant it. I tried to give her comfort and said,
"Thank you. And I want to thank you for your warm smiles each
time we came in here. It meant so much to us."

I was saying good-bye to another part of this hospital family.

When you began this journey you didn't know your way
around the hospital. Where is the cafeteria? Where is the family
resource center? Where is the gift shop? With time, you've
passed this information on to others who ask the same questions. In fact, you've joined a new family—the hospital family.
Courage increases for each one on this journey as encouragement passes from member to member.

Healing is in progress.

You need a God who can shape two fists of flesh into 75 to 100 billion nerve cells, each with as many as 10,000 connections to other nerve cells, place it in a skull, and call it a brain.

—Max Lucado

You're Not Alone

True survivors aren't found on a reality show on TV, but they are found in cancer families. These are the real life, true survivors. They've been shattered like broken glass on a tile floor and picked up with God's tender hands. Those jagged pieces fit into a new mosaic—the new normal.

Who are they? Some, like Hedy, have walked through the valley. Others have children still in treatment or in remission. All are surviving.

In April 1995, a jarring blast rocked Oklahoma City—the bombing of the Murrah Federal Building. Nearby, the First United Methodist Church suffered massive destruction, including its elaborate stained-glass windows. Now restored, one of the windows in the church's chapel was created from shards of stained glass. Worked into the breathtaking new window are these words: "The Lord takes broken pieces and by His love makes us whole."

Wherever you are on the journey, recently thrust into the tunnel, constantly thrown against the walls, or exiting into the sunlight, you can still choose to take the life God has given you and with passion and purpose complete what he has sent you here on earth to do.

Listen to Saint Paul's words in 2 Corinthians 4:8-9. He had an advanced degree in suffering: "*We are* hard-pressed on every side, yet not crushed; *we are* perplexed, but not in despair; persecuted; but not forsaken; struck down, but not destroyed."

"Will You Be Our Son's Pastor?"
—Chaplain Ward

I walked into the room; my eyes met the sixteen-year-old boy's indifferent glare. He was leaning back on his pillows propped up in bed and his arms were folded across his chest.

"Hi Randy, I'm Chaplain Ward."

"Uh, huh."

What a contrast to the previous week's meeting with his parents. Their eyes begged for help as they faced the life-ending illness of their only child. They struggled to hold onto their faith, and pleaded, "Will you be our son's pastor? He won't allow our pastor to come."

Randy allowed no one to get close to him. No one was going to talk about the dreadful diagnosis, and especially the probable outcome. How could I be his pastor? I prayed and then just showed up every day. The wall slowly came down, and another Randy appeared—a quiet-spirited, loving young man.

"What are your dreams, Randy?"

Immediately he answered, "Building and restoring race cars."

His face beamed as he described fluorescent paints and ear-splitting engine roars. In his hospital room, he couldn't rebuild race cars, but his heart opened to what he could do. As he walked his laps in the hall, God used him to brighten younger children's days. If he noticed a broken toy, he would ask if they wanted him to fix it. They were thrilled that a teenager took an interest in them.

> **In the End . . .**
>
> " . . . despite the chaos of the moment, no pain lasts forever and no evil triumphs in the end. Faith sees even the darkest deed of all history, the death of God's Son, as a necessary prelude to the brightest."
>
> —Philip Yancey,
> *Reaching for the Invisible God*

Our times together deepened, as his focus shifted from here to there to be with God. He started saying things like, "I've got some more people we need to pray for." But never for himself. He would also say, "I'm okay. Everything is going to be all right, and I'll be healed one way or the other—either here in remission or in heaven with no more cancer, chemo, and suffering."

Eventually, the time came; there were no more cures here. As I walked into his room, this time in ICU, there was that sixteen-year-old boy whose eyes had met me with indifference a month before; now he was glowing as he lay between this world and the next—the two worlds meeting in this room.

He whispered hoarsely, "Jesus is in the room, and everything's going to be okay." Then he fell back in a sedated sleep. Later he took his last breaths and whispered, "Shh . . . the angels are having a party. Can't you hear the music?"

Darkest Before the Dawn

In 1970, renowned preacher and author John Claypool tenderly held the hand of his ten-year-old daughter, Laura Lue, who was dying of leukemia. He said of this horrendous situation, " . . . I have no wings with which to fly or even legs on which to run— but listen, by the grace of God, I am still on my feet!" He continued, "This may not sound like much to you, but to me it is the most appropriate and most needful of all the gifts."

Several weeks after Laura Lue's death, exhausted but sleepless in the middle of the night, John wandered down to his study and opened a commentary to the familiar story of elderly Abraham and his long-awaited son, Isaac. He had preached that story many times, but that night, the Holy Spirit spoke to his broken heart with new insight. Did Abraham realize that Isaac had been given to him as a gift, not a possession—and given out of generous grace? In *Mending the Heart*, he said:

> I remember putting down the book that night as it dawned on me that Laura Lue had come into my life exactly as Isaac had come into Abraham's. I had never deserved her for a single day. She was not a possession to which I was entitled, but a gift by which I had been utterly blessed. And as that sense of her glowed in the darkness, I realized at that moment a choice stood before me. I could spend the rest of my life in anger and resentment because she had lived so short a time and so much

The Gift

"She was not a possession to which I was entitled, but a gift by which I had been utterly blessed."

—John Claypool
Mending the Heart

of her promise had been cut short, or I could spend the rest of my life in gratitude that she had ever lived at all and that I had the wonder of those ten grace-filled years. Jesus once promised that the Holy Spirit would help us to remember the things we should never forget, and that is exactly what happened to me that night.

> **God's Promise**
>
> But those who wait on the LORD shall renew *their* strength; They shall mount up with wings like eagles, They shall run and not be weary, They shall walk and not faint.
>
> —Isaiah 40:31

During this traumatic time in his family's life, John preached four gut-wrenching sermons, later published as a small but powerful book, *Tracks of a Fellow Struggler*, which still touches millions of strugglers today. John continued preaching, counseling and ministering as a "wounded healer" up to the end of his life. Even while suffering from cancer and recuperating from his second stem cell transplant in 2005, he sent handwritten notes and encouraging words to friends who were walking through their own deep waters. The woundedness that resulted from his daughter's death in 1970 still touched others in pain thirty-five years later. He joined Laura Lue in the fall of 2005.

Steps of Coping After a Loss

Caregivers focus all their energy on protecting and caring for their child. Where do they focus all that energy and compassion after their loss?

The answer is unique to each person. But a good place to start is with a prayer asking for the Lord's guidance: "Lord, please continue to heal and comfort our broken hearts, and to open new doors to help others."

So, how do we cope with the loss of those who die before we do? No matter the age, we're never fully prepared, and nothing makes sense during those dark days.

"I take one step forward and five back," a mom said.

Often our first response to death is childlike: We think, "He's gone forever!" or "That's not fair! He's mine!" Many adults relate to death in these terms. And many times we reel from one extreme to the other in our responses:

- Fight: "Just what on earth do you think you're doing, God!"
- Flight: "I give up. I can't feel you, God."

These are normal reactions. However, there's also a third possible reaction. This one is not controlled by your emotions like the first two, but it's controlled by your will—your choice to trust the "engineer" with the rest of the journey. That reaction demands that we step back and remember the truth that exists beyond our own feelings. That truth is expressed in this verse:

Therefore we do not lose heart. Even though our outward man is perishing, yet the inward *man* is being renewed day by day. For our light affliction, which is but for a moment, is working for us a far more exceeding *and* eternal weight of glory, while we do not look at the things which are seen, the things which are seen *are* temporary, but at the things which are not seen. (2 Cor. 4:16-18).

We can't have all the answers when we want them, but as we go through life day by day, many answers do appear. However, many times our actions must come before answers. Hold on to this truth—God has taken you through the first part of your life (the good ol' days), and he will be there for the rest of the journey (the new normal)—one step at a time.

Stages of Grief

These stages are a reminder that others have walked this road before you. Be alert though. Stages may not come in a neat order, and stages that you've already walked through may hit again—unexpectedly.

- Denial and isolation
- Anger
- Bargaining
- Depression—feelings of numbness, anger, and sadness may lurk underneath
- Acceptance

Of course, you need to be aware of your other children, the siblings walking alongside you through the grief process. Although you're grieving, they still need your presence and comfort. Furthermore, they may not experience the stages of grief in the order that you do. Allow them to grieve in their own way.

Someone said, "You alone can do your grief work, but you do not have to do it alone." God himself comes alongside us to help, and he sends fellow

Eternity
The seen world is temporary, but the unseen world is eternal.

travelers to do the same. They offer shining rays of hope—sometimes in unexpected ways.

Turning the Corner
—Hedy

I'd been wallowing in self-pity for a few weeks after Danielle's death—dragging through the fog, barely conscious of my two little girls, much less my husband. God had tried to comfort me, but I wasn't going to let him.

One night, I was out of the house grocery shopping, and at about 10:30, I called home.

"John, I've finished the shopping, but I'm not coming home now—I'm going to a movie."

"It's 10:30. You're going to go to a movie by yourself this late at night?"

"I'll be home later. I just need to be out longer. Are the kids in bed?"

"Yes, but be careful."

I decided to see *Spiderman 2*. That's what Danielle and I would have seen. She would have loved it. Popcorn in hand, I settled into the seat.

Then, in the middle of the movie—it hit. Spiderman had to make a decision. Give up his one true love and continue being Spiderman and helping mankind, or keep his girlfriend and give up being Spiderman. It was his agonizing choice.

Sacrifice

Surrendering sounds easy, but it isn't. God's Son laid down his life—for the good of all mankind. At any point, He could have called on thousands of angels to strike back or wield his own power to free himself of the blood-drenched cross. But He didn't. John 3:16 tells why.

My mind flashed back to the first of the week when I'd railed at God, "I'm going to cry all I want and you can't stop me. I know you're standing back waiting for me to slump in exhaustion, but instead I'm going shopping." (And to the movies!)

Suddenly, I felt like God was saying, "Spiderman had a decision and you do too. Let go of your daughter, for the good of mankind—for your other daughters, husband, mankind. . . ."

Sitting in the movie theater I silently shouted at God, "NO! I don't want to do that, God. I want to hold on to the grief!"

But then I realized that it was a choice, and I had to make it . . . and it was time. Driving home, peace invaded my car.

As I walked into my house, John smiled and surrounded me in his arms. "You okay?" he whispered in my ear.

I leaned against his shoulder and said, "I will be."

Struck Down, But Not Destroyed

In the mid-nineties, Mickey and Jenny's toddler, Melody, began limping. After extensive tests, the diagnosis: a stroke. Even though they were told not to worry, they pushed for further tests. Second diagnosis: brain tumor. Prognosis: two months to live.

Days became months as surgery, chemo, infections, remission, aneurism, more surgeries, another poor prognosis, and shunts filled their lives. "Our world turned upside-down," said Jenny.

Mickey added, "I remember lying on the floor next to her crib, and just crying, 'Why are you doing this?'"

Other parts of their life crumbled, including losing their house, cars, and jobs—one right after the other. The medical insurance company they were using went out of business and they frantically searched for a new medical plan.

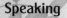

Speaking

God's word is powerful. He spoke the universe into existence, and his Word (the Bible) still speaks today—especially in your up-side-down world.

Mickey continued, "Everything was falling apart, and one night we'd been yelling at each other—completely not like our usual personalities—and all of a sudden, God spoke in my heart. 'Stop! You're giving Satan the glory in your reactions, not Me. I want you to worship and glorify Me, not Satan.' I grabbed Jenny's hand and told her what I was feeling. We fell to the floor and prayed, and his peace just poured over us, even joy for the first time. Do you know what Melody means? Song of joy. The peace we felt was purely mercy on God's behalf. The Holy Spirit guided us each day, and things haven't been the same since. Melody wasn't healed overnight, but she has steadily improved, and now she's a precious eleven-year-old with a big smile."

"But the thing is," Jenny added, "we were to praise and trust him no matter what. If she's healed here on earth or not. We are so thankful she's better, but the scary part is when we look back and remember where we were in that spiritual darkness."

She flipped through the pages of her well-marked Bible and said, "Here are the verses that kept us going: 'Seeing then that we have a great High Priest who has passed through the heavens, Jesus the Son of God, let us hold fast *our* confession. For we do not have a High Priest who cannot sympathize with our weaknesses, but was in all *points* tempted as *we are*, yet without sin. Let us therefore come boldly to the throne of grace, that we may obtain mercy and find grace to help in time of need'" (Heb. 4:14-16).

Mickey said, "That's just what I'd tell anyone going through this. Fall on your knees. He's there."

Mickey and Jenny were not alone in the chaos. Their friend, Jay, walked closely with them. Jay met with Mickey every Saturday morning to talk and pray. One night, Mickey called Jay to say the doctors didn't expect Melody to live through the night. During the night Jay woke up with a song playing in his mind. He wrote down the words.

> Some years ago,
> You loaned Your love to me
> You sang a song, the sweetest melody
> The years to come I thought were mine to keep
> Now all I have is a melody in my sleep
> The Lord gives and the Lord taketh away
> With tender care, He hides the sun at the
>   end of every day
> The promise of a sunrise is what gets us
>   through the night
> All I can do is trust in Him
> All I can do is wait for the light.
> (Music and words by Jay Young, first two verses)

Miraculously, Melody made it through all the years of surgery and treatments. She's a normal, happy girl today. God brings others alongside to give you hope and courage. And he is with you in the chaos—you're not alone.

We do not serve a distant god who spouts encouraging clichés from the sideline. Instead, he enters into our suffering . . . God will never leave us on our own.

—Rick Warren, *The Purpose Driven Life:
What On Earth Am I Here For?*

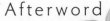

Preparing for the Journey

Life on planet earth is a journey. Somehow we think that journey should always be smooth. We'll accept a *few* bumps, but we certainly don't expect to be plunged into fearful tunnels. When that happens, we reel in the darkness and want answers—and solutions. Others want to give us those answers and help us see solutions. However, many times the answers don't come quickly, but the waiting pulls us to him.

Bearing Up
—Elizabeth

I've heard so often from people that God doesn't give us more than we can bear. But I have found that's wrong. This is more than I can handle, it's more than I can bear. We are facing the possible death of our child.

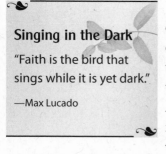

Singing in the Dark

"Faith is the bird that sings while it is yet dark."

—Max Lucado

On a daily basis, we are facing our son's pain and discomfort—and often we are the ones who give him that pain by administering drugs and treatments that cause him to feel bad. And every week he develops some new side effect and we don't know which drug is causing it.

Every Friday we have to say, "We're going to the hospital," which entails scary moments and pain. We can't let him drink water on these mornings, and so he goes all Thursday night and Friday morning without even the comfort of a sippy cup of milk.

So this is way more than any of us can bear. But God IS giving us the strength to LEARN how to bear it. God has allowed all of this to happen—and I'm not sure why yet. It may take me years to come to grips with it and years to forgive him. But he'll see us through. And I believe that. So many people have shared with me the good things that have happened in their lives as a result of Adam getting sick. I'm glad there is fruit from this horrible situation.

His Promise

Elizabeth in California, Hedy in Georgia, and all the other precious families coast to coast who have shared their stories in this book have experienced that God never leaves us alone. As the second verse of this old hymn states, "Tho' all around me is darkness, Earthly joys all flown; My Savior whispers His promise, Never to leave me alone." That's God's promise.

No, Never Alone
(19th Century song, Anonymous)

I've seen the lightning flashing,
I've heard the thunder roll,
I've felt sin's breakers dashing,
Which almost conquered my soul;
I've heard the voice of my Savior
Bidding me still to fight on;
He promised never to leave me,
Never to leave me alone.

When in affliction's valley
I tread the road of care,
My Savior helps me to carry
The cross so heavy to bear;
Tho' all around me is darkness,
Earthly joys all flown;
My Savior whispers His promise,
Never to leave me alone.

You're never alone.

Resources

You-niquely Made Personality Study

U sing the You-niquely Made Personality Study can help you understand and appreciate family, friends, and medical staff—all uniquely made. Jot notes to jog your memory of how to best meet their needs—and your needs also.

Vibrant Yellow's sunshine can brighten your day, but too much can drain you dry. Sensitive Blue's rain clouds create beauty, but too many can be depressing. Determined Red's instructions are helpful, but can be overbearing. Calm Green's steadfast roots grow deep, but can be unmovable. This resource should help you see the bright side of each color's personality and deal with each color's frailties.

Remember that each color and combination (blend) has strengths and weaknesses. Some move, eat, and speak slowly, some fast. Some need people around constantly; others want to be alone. To some, everything is either right or wrong; others go with the flow.

Each color has different coping skills. The Yellow parent hits the wall but bounces back quickly and says, "Don't be so negative." The opposite Blue parent wants all the information given correctly, and makes decisions slowly and thoroughly. "You can't make that decision off the top of your head," she says. The Red parent doesn't want details, rabbit trails, or an idea that fails: "We're going to beat this!" The opposite Green parent goes with the flow (as much as possible), listens, and when pressed to give an opinion, says, "Whatever they think is best."

Different factors drain and fill their emotional tanks. Developing appreciation for each gene color will improve your communication and relationships. Appreciation prevents you from taking anyone for granted. God designed us to communicate effectively with others and with him. He gave us his Designer genes! King David said, "For You formed my inward parts; You covered me in my mother's womb. I will praise You, for I am fearfully *and* wonderfully made; Marvelous are Your works, And *that* my soul knows very well" (Ps. 139:13-14).

Vibrant Yellows

You hear Yellows before you see them—and continue to hear them and hear them and hear them. Full of energy, they bounce into rooms, eyes sparkling, and wearing a perpetual smile. They pounce and hug anyone in reach. They make Tigger look passive.

To a Yellow, everyone is a best friend. They make those friends in elevators, standing in line at the grocery store, or answering a telemarketer's questions. Seldom wanting to be alone, they need "people fixes" often.

Yellows begin many things, but they finish few. They constantly hear the following refrains:

- "How can you live in all that clutter?"
- "Where are your keys?"
- "You got lost where? Again?"

What drains their emotional tanks? Being alone and having to finish anything carefully (not simply slapping it together).

How do they react when their emotional tanks register empty? They talk more and louder. (Their opposites—the Blues can't imagine that Yellows can talk more or louder). If that doesn't work, they get totally quiet, and everyone says, "What's wrong with her, she's so quiet?"

How do you fill Yellow's emotional tank? You fill it with people—giving them time, talk, and touch (many hugs). You can also help them with organization.

So, how do Yellows fill others' tanks? They brighten a room. We can all use the warmth they give, especially on dreary days.

Snapshot: When Yellow Brightened a Dreary Day

As Diane walked wearily from the parking garage to the hospital, her mind was preoccupied with her daughter's serious surgery.

"Well, hi there!" a tiny voice interrupted.

She looked around, then down. There stood a small, smiling boy. His father stood behind him, locking the car.

"Hi there," Diane replied.

"What you doin' here?"

"I'm visiting my daughter. She's sick."

"I'm gonna see my nana," the boy said and rapidly shot the details.

His father sighed and said, "Son, leave the lady alone."

"Oh, that's okay."

The boy continued his story, as the father repeated, "Son, leave the lady alone."

To please the dad, Diane said, "I need to get on in. You have a good day." A few seconds later Diane was approaching the hospital door.

"Well, hi there," she heard the same boy say to a lady getting out of her car. "What you doin' here?" And his father repeating again, "Son leave the lady alone." Inside the hospital, as she headed down the gray corridor, Diane smiled. "Thank you, Lord. I really needed that little ray of sunshine!"

Helpful Hints if You're a Yellow

Yellows have trouble focusing, especially on things they don't want to do. Result? Things pile up and they feel overwhelmed. Yellows, focus on the first and most important task you need to do. Finish that before you go to the second. To do that, you may need to take small bites of the elephant.

The task you've been putting off may look like an elephant, so remember this: you can't eat an elephant at one sitting. In the same way, you can't complete a huge task quickly. You have to take small bites—tackle small parts of the job. Here's a helpful hint if you find you can't stay at a task for a long time. Set a timer for fifteen minutes. You can do almost anything for that length of time. Take small bites; do parts of a big task, and be thankful for what you accomplish.

Now what's that task you've put off? Cleaning a bathroom floor covered with dirty clothes and wet towels? Filing hospital papers and overdue bills? Finding your keys—again? Get started—not after one more computer game, telephone call, or e-mail excuse.

If you're a Yellow, you have to take the time to make a home for everything. Once you accomplish that task and put things back in their place each time, it will become a habit. You'll put the dirty clothes and towels in the hamper, the mail in a certain stack (a shoebox will work),

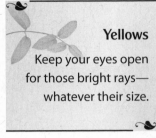

Yellows
Keep your eyes open for those bright rays—whatever their size.

and the keys back on the hook. Surprisingly, you'll be able to find items when you need them and save valuable time and frustration. Blues do all of this instinctively.

Give Thanks for Yellows

Who are the Yellows in your life? Jot down their names and tell them thanks—they'll probably do even more. Even weary Yellows spread sunshine. Here are a few things to be thankful for in the Yellows you know:

- Continual, contagious smile
- Hugs
- Friendliness—especially important to others who may be shy
- High energy level when others are winding down
- Clicks with children

Be thankful for those lights shining in the darkness.

Sensitive Blues

You've met the high-energy, talkative, outgoing Yellows. They multitask, start many projects, and finish few. Although their roller-coaster emotions zoom from tears to laughter, they still "go with the flow" as situations change. They see their glass at least half-full or overflowing as they spread their optimistic sunshine.

Who are the Blues? In contrast to the Yellows, they're low-energy, quiet introverts. They do one thing at a time, slowly, and stay with it until it's completed perfectly. Their emotions, accompanied by sighing, register on two levels—deep and deeper. Blues don't like to go with the flow because transitions are traumatic. They need time to process the changes, and the new cancer journey is packed with overwhelming transitions.

They see their glass half-empty—and draining. "Our half-empty glass is how the world really is," said a Blue. "At least we see things in an objective way."

We need Blue's devotion to detail, to jobs done well—such as balancing the checkbook to the penny—even if it takes them hours to do so. (Yellows guesstimate with checkbooks.) Blues correctly fill out hospital papers and meticulously place them in folders. Blues seriously think through situations, ponder, and in time give you their answer. People turn to them because they know Blues genuinely care. They read people well but sometimes read into situations more than is there.

When overwhelmed in a crisis, pushed to hurry up, or deprived of time alone, their emotional tank empties rapidly. They may become worn out or depressed, or they may simply shut down. As things build inside, eventually an explosion may happen, leaving people confused. "What's wrong with her? She never acts like that, she's usually so quiet." If you're a Blue, you need to share what's going on. Let people know how you feel. No one can read your mind.

How do you fill Blue's emotional tank? Give them lots of solitary time in a space of their own—away from crowds and noise—so they can process information. They live by their own time schedule and their way of doing things. Since transitions are traumatic, alert them to coming changes and give them time to adjust.

Which ones usually marry each other? Many times, it is the opposite Yellows and Blues. Notice the totally different needs in Yellows and Blues? What helps one probably won't help the other; communication is desperately needed.

While going through the tunnel, we especially need Blue's sympathy, hugs, and organizational skills.

Snapshot: Blue to the Rescue

"How's your wife doing?" Yellow Roy's voice boomed across the room.

"I got her home from the hospital Wednesday," the weary husband answered.

Roy slapped him on the back. "Well, that's great," he said while looking around the room.

The husband continued, "But I'm not sure where we go from here—"

"Uh huh," Roy replied as he spotted his next encounter and headed off, adding his traditional, "I'll be praying for you."

That's the picture. Yellow playing Duck, Duck, Goose, touching people as he continued in circles, not recognizing the deep need standing before him.

Then up walked Blue Dave, slipping his arm around the weary husband's shoulder. "Claude, how's Jenny doing?"

As Claude related the last week's journey and the uncertainty of the tomorrows, Dave listened. He made Claude feel as if he were the only person in the room.

Blues

Blues quietly wrap around hurting people, giving support.

"I'm so sorry you're going through this. May I come by this afternoon and we'll talk?

Noticing Claude's eyes brim with tears, Dave continued, "Can I pray with you right now?"

Helpful Hints if You're a Blue

Life is a process, not perfection. Your halfway effort will be better than almost everyone else's best tries, so don't procrastinate because you feel you have to attempt perfection.

Appreciate all that the different colors have to offer.

You have deep feelings for others and take on their hurts, especially on this difficult journey. However, you may feel that optimistic Yellows aren't serious enough, driven Reds don't care enough, and passive Greens don't show enough emotion.

Pray for acceptance and appreciation of others. We're all in this together and desperately need each other.

Give Thanks for Blues

Who are they in your life? Jot down names and tell them thanks. They will appreciate your thoughtfulness. Here are a few things to be thankful for in the Blues you know:

- Feels deeply
- Supports friends no matter what
- Organizes everything
- Manages money (this journey needs that quality)
- Analyzes decisions carefully

Be thankful for sensitive Blue genes.

Determined Reds!

Fasten your seatbelt—here come the Reds. They know what needs to be done, how to do it, and want it done now. They demand the bottom line (of whatever is happening) and don't care about details. Just get it done, then move on to the next task.

Reds persevere no matter the obstacles and can't understand why everyone else doesn't do the same. "I walked around on a broken leg for a week, she's complaining about a sprained ankle," stated a Red.

Two Reds together? They both think they're right. In a faceoff, they wait for the other to realize it.

"You should have seen the standoff between my child and her first oncologist. I wasn't sure which one would win. It changed from day to day," said a mom.

They keep people's feet to the fire, not cutting them slack while working circles around everyone. So do they need their emotional tanks filled? Yes, whether they realize it or not. You can tell when they're on empty; they get louder and more demanding. If that doesn't work, they get totally quiet—everyone then waits for the other shoe to drop.

How do you fill a Red's tank? Give them appreciation for what they do—that's how they show love. Saying something like, "Thanks for all your hard work getting this information and getting the job done" is music to their ears.

Also, don't give them details, stay off rabbit trails, and simply give the bottom line.

When the going gets rough, or if you simply need a guide, you need a Red.

Snapshot: A Trip to NYC

At a NYC hotel, a Red mom unpacked suitcases and said to her husband and daughter (both Blue-Greens), "I've made an agenda so we can make the best use of our time."

Dad and daughter smiled and rolled their eyes at each other.

"Mom, can I just rest for a few minutes?" moaned the teenager.

"We don't want to waste this weekend in the room."

"Do we have to walk everywhere?"

"Of course not. The subway's right across the street. Let's go."

The three headed out, agenda clutched in mom's hand. She walked briskly and spoke into the air, "Isn't this great!" Her husband and daughter knew the answer they were to give but were busy trying to keep up the pace.

They raced down steep stairs leading to the subway. Mom stopped to check the subway map.

"Why do you want to look at this? You've got it all planned out," said her husband.

"It's fun to see where we are on the map and where we're going." She traced her finger along the color-coded routes. "Let's try this other line and see if we can cut off some stops."

"Mom, we're gonna get lost."

"Of course we won't. Besides, this is an adventure."

"Does the adventure include going back to the room this afternoon?"

"You really want to do that?"

"Can't I just rest for a little while?"

"OK, but you'll miss all the afternoon— "

"That's okay, Mom."

Backtracking to the hotel, daughter was left to rest and read. She was happy.

Mom hit the pavement in full stride, checking off her list. She was happy.

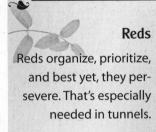

Reds

Reds organize, prioritize, and best yet, they persevere. That's especially needed in tunnels.

Dad attempted keeping up with mom. We think he was happy, but we know he was exhausted.

Back home, two days later, mom announced, "Wasn't that a great trip!"

"Uh huh," they answered.

Two months later, dad and daughter looked through the trip pictures again, "You know, that was fun," said dad.

"Yeah, but don't tell Mom."

Both smiled and rolled their eyes.

Helpful Hints if You're a Red

Stop, look, and listen:

- Stop—or at least slow down. You're used to telling others to stop, now do so yourself.
- Look—at others in the eye, not above their shoulder or at your watch.
- Listen—to what others say.

Keep your opinions (how they could do things better) to yourself, unless asked. When you do speak the truth, do it in love. Be tactfully truthful.

Give your time, attention, and encouragement as gifts to others. They respect your opinion, especially if you've done the previous three steps.

Give Thanks for Reds

Who are they in your life? Jot down names and tell them thanks—if you can catch them. Here are a few things to be thankful for in the Reds you know:

- High energy, when others wind down
- Objectively sees the big picture—what needs to be done and how to do it—give the bottom line
- Tenaciously perseveres until a task is complete
- Keeps self and others on task (holds their feet to the fire)
- Excels in a crisis ("He lives for times like this," is usually said of a Red)

Be thankful for those who shout, "Stop. I can help."

Calm Greens

Now sit back and relax. Can you hear the soothing sound of a porch swing clicking back and forth and back and forth and. . . . That's like the go-with-the-flow, predictable Greens. Emotionally, they have no highs and no lows. They're great in a crisis. They get along with almost everyone.

Greens go through life in slow motion—whether walking, talking, or eating. This pace drives Reds crazy. "When I tell her to hurry, she slows down!"

Reds and Greens are two more opposites who may end up marrying each other.

Greens don't demand attention so they can be easily overlooked. Of growing up in a household with more demanding siblings, a Green once said, "I felt invisible at the dinner table with my two brothers who hogged all the attention."

Teachers may not remember the names of their Green students because they're busy keeping up with the Reds and Yellows that are bouncing around the room.

Green's emotional tank drains slowly, but it does drain—especially when alone time becomes packed with people and activities. They become quieter, finally digging in their heels, not budging. Since they've gone along with everyone before, people are surprised at this reaction. "I told him we're going out to dinner, and he just sat there reading the paper. He wouldn't move!" stated a Red wife.

How do you fill these easygoing emotional tanks?

"You mean he really needs something?" asked his wife.

Yes, and since Greens don't demand attention, hearing their name or appreciation for what they've done will fill their tanks quickly.

Remember their low energy level; they live for a good nap. Let them have one.

Greens are low-key, undemanding children who passively enter a low-key, undemanding adulthood.

Snapshot: Teacher's Lounge, 1984

"I'm so relieved they didn't laugh him off the stage." My teacher colleague was telling us about the speaker at her son's Ivy League college graduation that past weekend. "I watched as he sauntered up to the podium, smiled at the graduating class, and then he started singing: 'It's a beautiful day in the neighborhood. . . .'

"I held my breath, as those unresponsive seniors stared silently at the stage. Then, during the song, they slowly melted into swaying three-year-olds leaning forward on their folding chairs. They even joined in singing his song. He had them in the palm of his hand. I can't remember what all he said, just how he

> **Greens**
>
> Greens give uncondi-tional love, accepting you just as you are.

said it. Then as he closed, they jumped to their feet clapping, whistling, and the girls rushed the stage shoving programs for his autograph. They yelled, 'Remember, me?' I guess they thought he'd seen them through the TV set years ago." All of us smiled and nodded as she continued.

"And, I loved all those sophisticated seniors shouting, 'Get my picture with my best friend, Mr. Rogers.' He just patiently stood there smiling with those kids as flashbulbs kept going off."

As a young child, extremely shy Fred Rogers was encouraged by his Grandfather McFeely. Fred became the nationally famous Mr. Rogers—encouraging generations through unconditional love.

Helpful Hints if You're a Green

Procrastination may be a familiar problem to you. Yellows procrastinate because they take on too much; Greens procrastinate because they use lack of energy as their excuse. Like Yellows, you need to take small bites of the elephant (see the helpful hints for Yellows). Greens need to focus, especially to finish tasks.

You should also speak up and give feedback. Don't be prideful saying, "Hum, no one knows what I'm thinking." It's counterproductive. Also, others need your input to help make decisions. You have a balanced outlook. Yes, even Reds need it.

Give Thanks for Greens

Who are they in your life? Jot down names and be sure to thank them—by name. Here are a few things to be thankful for in the Greens you know:

- Sits and listens, doesn't interrupt
- Goes with the flow; acts rather than react
- Creates calmness in crisis
- Reliable
- Sees things objectively

Be thankful for relaxed Green genes.

Ways We Give and Receive Love

Dovetailing with color-coded personalities is the understanding of how others give and receive love, Gary Chapman explains in his Five Love Languages book series. Who needs what in your family to refill those empty emotional tanks?

According to Chapman, love is given and received in five primary languages. These are some examples of what someone who gives and receives in each love language would express:

- **Talk.** "Let me hear something positive. I need to know I'm doing something right."
- **Touch.** Babies thrive on it; children feel special with it; teens may not acknowledge it, but desire a passing nudge; adults sometimes admit, "I just need a hug."
- **Time.** "Just sit down and spend time with me. Don't be glancing at your watch."
- **Gifts.** "I can't believe my sister gave me a little shell from last summer's trip. And you know, gifts don't have to cost anything—it's enough that someone thinks about me in a tangible way. I can glance at the shell and relive the moment for a long time."

- **Deeds.** "OK, so you say, 'I love you,' a lot. When you pick your wet towels off the floor and hang them up, I'll know you mean it. Actions speak louder than words."

"My wife 'speaks' three of the love languages, and I speak the other two. Amazing we communicate at all," a husband said and laughed.

Which languages are important to you? How about others in your family? Talk it over and each week have everyone write down one thing they need. As the family meets each other's emotional needs, everyone wins. Pray for the willingness and follow-through to give these gifts—in and out of the tunnel.

Chapman's books have strengthened families and influenced countless relationships. More information on his books is given in the Bibliography.

Organizations & Websites

The following associations and organizations are helpful sources of additional information for your journey.

American Cancer Society (ACS)
www.cancer.org
Dedicated to helping everyone who faces cancer through research, patient services, early detection, treatment, and education. Find information for patients, family,

American Childhood Cancer Organization
www.acco.org
ACCO's mission is to provide information and awareness for children and adolescents with cancer and their families, to advocate for their needs, and to support research so every child survives and leads a long healthy life. This organization was formerly known as the Candlelighters Childhood Cancer Foundation.

Association of Cancer Online Resources (ACOR)
www.acor.org/ped-onc
Resources, web links, and references for parents, friends, and families of children who have or had childhood cancer.

CareFlash
www.careflash.com
Free, personal web pages helping families and friends communicate.

CarePages
www.carepages.com
Free, personal, and private web pages that help family and friends communicate when someone is receiving care.

CaringBridge
www.caringbridge.org
Offers free, easy-to-create websites that help connect friends and family when they need it most.

Children's Cancer Association
www.childrenscancerassociation.org
CCA is composed of parents, medical professionals, community leaders, and individuals; and provides service to seriously ill children and their families over 22,800 times a year.

Cure Search for Children's Cancer
www.curesearch.org
Unites the world's largest childhood cancer research organizations,

the Children's Oncology Group (COG) and the National Childhood Cancer Foundation. Information on support systems and camps across the country.

The Leukemia and Lymphoma Society
www.lls.org
Financial assistance and consultation services for referrals to other means of local support. Educational materials for parents and family members through local chapters and the home office.

National Cancer Institute
www.cancer.gov
Provides comprehensive information about diagnoses, statistics, research, clinical trials, and news.

The National Children's Cancer Society
www.nationalchildrenscancersociety.org
Independent, national organization provides a broad range of services, including financial and in-kind assistance, advocacy, support services, and education and prevention programs.

The Neuroblastoma Children's Cancer Society (NCCS)
www.neuroblastomacancer.org
Serves as advocates for the children who suffer from neuroblastoma and as a support center for their families. Offers the Wall of Fame, educational materials, and more.

The Never Ending Squirrel Tale
www.squirreltales.com
This upbeat and encouraging site was started by a Montana woman, Debby Caron, whose friend's daughter had cancer. The site provides information for parents of children with cancer as well as resources and communities. The website contains fact sheets, personal stories, spiritual inspiration sections, bulletin boards, scrapbooks, newsletters, articles, practical tips, and links to other resources.

Pediatric Brain Tumor Foundation of the United States
www.pbtfus.org
Supporting the search for the cause and cure of childhood brain tumors through research. See upcoming events for families & survivors in your area.

Pediatric Oncology Resource Center
www.ped-onc.org
Resources and information for parents of children with cancer, by parents of children with cancer.

Ronald McDonald House Charities
rmhc.org
Many major cities have these facilities where out-of-town families can stay while their children are being treated for a serious illness. Room rates are economical, and a social worker may be able to help locate one.

Recommended Inspirational Reading

In addition to the recommended books I mention throughout this book, I also recommend reading the following books for hope and comfort.

Guthrie, Nancy. *The One Year Book of Hope.* Wheaton, IL: Tyndale House, 2005.

Littauer, Florence. *Silver Linings: Breaking through the Clouds of Depression.* Birmingham, AL: New Hope Publishers, 2006.

Lotz, Ann Graham. *Why? Trusting God When You don't Understand.* Nashville: W Publishing, 2004.

Morgan, Robert J. *Red Sea Rules: The Same God Who Led You in Will Lead You Out.* Nashville: Thomas Nelson Books, 2001. Ten God-given strategies for difficult times.

MacLellan, Scott Neil. *Amanda's Gift: One Family's Journey Through the Maze of Serious Childhood Illness.* Roswell, GA: Health Awareness Communication, 1999.

Tucker, Sherry. *Unfinished Love: Walking by Faith through Pediatric Cancer.* VMI Publishers, 2008. givinghopethroughfaith.org

Yancey, Philip. *PRAYER: Does It Make Any Difference?* Grand Rapids, MI: Zondervan, 2006.

Bibliography

The following books were used in developing the information in this book. I highly recommend reading them.

Chapter 2

Corrie ten Boom knew dark tunnels intimately. Fifty-something Corrie, her frail older sister Betsy, and their elderly father were arrested in Amsterdam by the Gestapo for hiding Jewish neighbors. They were interrogated, crammed into empty cattle cars, and endured brutal concentration camps, all the while trusting the "engineer" —God. Her story of his daily presence in her life brings hope in the midst of unbearable pain as described in *The Hiding Place* (Bantam 1984).

Chapter 7

Brand, Dr. Paul and Philip Yancey. *In His Image.* Grand Rapids, MI: Zondervan, 1987.

Chapman, Gary. *The Five Love Languages of God.* Chicago: Northfield Publishing, 2002.

Meinders, Le Donna. *Angel Hugs for Cancer Patients: Heavenly Embraces for Everyday Life.* St. Louis, MO: Chalice Press, 2002.

Chapter 8

Kent, Carol. *When I Lay My Isaac Down: Unshakable Faith in Unthinkable Circumstances.* Colorado Springs, CO: Navpress, 2004.

Robinson, Barbara. *Best Christmas Pageant Ever.* New York: HarpCollins, 1972.

Chapter 12

Claypool, John R. *Tracks of a Fellow Struggler: Living and Growing through Grief.* Harrisburg, PA: Morehouse, 2003.

Claypool, John R. *Mending the Heart.* Lanham, MD: Rowman & Littlefield, 1999.

Yancey, Philip. *Reaching for the Invisible God: What Can We Expect to Find?* Grand Rapids, MI: Zondervan, 2000.

Afterwords

Lucado, Max. *God Came Near,* Nashville: Thomas Nelson, 2004.

Warren, Rick. *The Purpose Driven Life: What On Earth Am I Here For?* Grand Rapids: Zonndervan, 2002.

Resource One

Chapman, Gary. *The Five Love Languages: How to Express Heartfelt Commitment to Your Mate.* Chicago: Northfield Press, 2004.

Chapman, Gary. *The Five Love Languages of Teens.* Chicago: Northfield Press, 2005.

Chapman, Gary and Ross Campbell. *The Five Love Languages of Children.* Chicago: Northfield Press, 2005.

Scripture Reference

215

Index

About the Authors

Lynda T. Young, MRE, M.Ed, is the cofounder of Kindred Spirits International whose outreaches include children's hospitals and the Amani ya Juu, refugee women's mission in Kenya. She is a writer, national speaker, and has done hospital volunteer work at Children's Healthcare of Atlanta. She authored the You Are Not Alone book series, which includes Hope for Families of Children with Cancer, Hope for Families of Children with Congenital Heart Defects, and Hope for Families of Children on the Autistic Spectrum. Her husband, Dr. John L.Young, a professor at Emory University, has been in cancer research for over forty years. They are blessed with four children, eleven grandchildren, and four great-grandchildren.

Chaplain Johnnathan R. Ward, MDIV, is a senior staff chaplain with Children's Healthcare of Atlanta, Aflac Cancer Center and Blood Disorders Service, Atlanta, GA. He has walked daily in the trenches with children and families as they journey the difficult stages of a cancer diagnosis. He understands the exceptional challenges that families face and the spiritual support so needed. As the coordinator for wellness activities in the Aflac Cancer Center at Egleston, Johnnathan designs and leads staff support programs, retreats, and workshops. These programs aid in the retention of staff and help to lessen the impact of "compassion fatigue." He is a much sought after workshop and retreat leader dealing with grief, caring for the caregiver, and remembering your child through rituals. Johnnathan has served as a chaplain in the hospital, military, and substance abuse environments. He has served as a pastor, missionary in Africa, and coordinator for the State of Georgia's Responsible Fatherhood Program. He seeks to live by the spiritual teaching, "Do unto others as you would have them do unto you." He is married to Vashti Maharaj-Ward for seventeen wonderful years and they have two children, Shivani and Sahadev.

You Are Not Alone!

Lynda Young Shares with Parents, Families, Friends

Lynda Young speaks from her heart and touches thousands with the clear message that You Are Not Alone! With energy, passion and extensive experience, she travels the journey with families, caregivers, and caring friends of children who are hurting.

Lynda brings hope and calm in the midst of distress and suffering. Come along with Lynda as she brings clarity of what IS possible during the journey and how to actively contribute in new ways that brings comfort to all involved. Her topics include . . .

I'm Sorry to Tell You This, Your Child Has...
Journeying along with families who hear the news, and need to understand and cope with the 'new normal.'

When Your Emotional Tank Registers Empty
Effective communication tools during stressful situations.

Siblings: the Invisible Ones
Meeting the needs of the "well" one.

"Root Wrapping"—
Just as gigantic Redwoods intertwine their shallow roots, strengthening them during severe storms, so we as humans "root wrap" with others during storms in our lives. We help the hurting.

Bring Lynda Young to your church groups,
retreats, and conferences to speak with families,
caregiver, church leadership, and counselors.

For more information visit
www.HopeforFamiliesOnline.com